The Seven Spiritual Laws of Yoga

A Practical Guide to Healing Body, Mind, and Spirit

Deepak Chopra, M.D.

David Simon, M.D.

WILEY

John Wiley & Sons, Inc.

Published by John Wiley & Sons, Inc., Hoboken, New Jersey
Published simultaneously in Canada

Design and Production by Navta Associates, Inc.

Photography is by Omry Reznick Photography. The models used in the photos are: Claire Diab, Michael Fukumura, Roger Gabriel, and Pam Simon.

For general information about our other products and services, please contact our Customer Care Department within the United States at (800) 762-2974, outside the United States at (317) 572-3993 or fax (317) 572-4002.

Wiley also publishes its books in a variety of electronic formats. Some content that appears in print may not be available in electronic books. For more information about Wiley products, visit our web site at www.wiley.com.

Library of Congress Cataloging-in-Publication Data:

Chopra, Deepak.
   The seven spiritual laws of yoga : a practical guide to healing body, mind, and spirit / Deepak Chopra, David Simon.
      p. cm.
   Includes bibliographical references and index.
   ISBN-13 978-0-471-64764-5 (cloth)
   ISBN-10 0-471-64764-0 (cloth)
   ISBN-13 978-0-471-73627-1 (paper)
   ISBN-10 0-471-73627-9 (paper)
   1. Yoga, Râaja—Popular works. 2. Health—Popular works. 3. Mind and body—Popular works. I. Simon, David. II. Title.
   RA781.7.C4798   2004
   294.5'436—dc22
                                                              2004005665

Printed in the United States of America

10 9 8 7 6 5

This book is dedicated
to seekers of unity across time and space

Contents

Preface
The Four Yogas

Often one goes for one thing and finds another.
—Neem Karoli Baba

The word *yoga* is related to the English word *yoke*.
Yoga is the union of body, mind, and spirit—the
union of your individuality with the divine intelligence
that orchestrates the universe. Yoga is a state of being in
which the elements and forces that comprise your biological organism are in harmonious interaction with the elements of the cosmos. Established in this state, you will
experience enhanced emotional, psychological, and spiritual well-being and will increasingly notice the spontaneous fulfillment of your desires. In yoga—in union with
spirit—your desires and the desires of nature are one. As
you participate in the process of creativity along with the
infinite being, your worries fall away and you feel a sense

of lightheartedness and joy. There is a spontaneous blossoming of intuition, insight, imagination, creativity,
meaning, and purpose. You make correct choices that
benefit not only you but also everyone affected by your
choices. When in the book of Matthew Jesus says, "My
yoke is easy, and my burden is light," he is expressing the
core principle of yoga. His intelligence is aligned with
cosmic intelligence, his will with divine will.

Traditionally, there are four forms of yoga: *Gyan, Bhakti,
Karma,* and *Raja.* Gyan yoga is the yoga of understanding.
The yoga of understanding is also the yoga of science.
(Science is after all, the knowledge of nature's laws.)
The laws of nature are God's thoughts. Science is God
explaining God to God through a human nervous system.
Science is not an enemy of spiritual awakening but rather
a potentially helpful friend. Today's science reveals to us
the mysterious nonlocal domain where everything is
instantly correlated with everything else—where time,
space, matter, energy, and information resolve into a field
of pure potentiality. This is the realm where the immeasurable potential of all that was, all that is, and all that will
be manifests and differentiates into the seer and the
scenery, the observer and the observed, the knower and
the known.

  The yoga of understanding has been referred to in the
Upanishads as the "razor's edge," and we are cautioned to
tread carefully on this path. As we gain understanding of
the laws of nature, we run the risk of arrogance. Arrogance
inflates the ego, and the ego overshadows the spirit. The
original sincere quest for discovery leads to an alienation
from the very source with which intimacy was sought.

Truly great scientists are known for their humility, for even as they explore and unravel the secrets of the unknown, the unknown looms larger and becomes ever more mysterious. Humility leads to wonder, which leads to innocence. The return of innocence invites us to enter the luminous mystery of life and surrender to it.

The yoga of knowledge can be a wonderful path if we are mature enough to understand that there are seductive temptations that may entrap us for a while in diversions of the intellect.

The second yoga is Bhakti—the yoga of love and devotion. Bhakti is love of God but also the expression and blossoming of love in all your relationships. The divine light of God resides in all that is alive, or for that matter, even that which we consider inanimate. Through our relationships with others, we discover our higher self. As we embark on this journey, we may go through stages of attraction, infatuation, communion, intimacy, surrender, passion and ecstasy until ultimately we once again arrive at the source of love and the source of life.

The yoga of love is a wonderful path, but we must not confuse love with self-absorption, self-importance, or self-pity. If you pay attention to love, think about love, express love, respond to gestures of love, and make love the basis for all your choices, then you are practicing Bhakti yoga, the yoga of love.

The third yoga is referred to as Karma yoga. The ultimate expression of Karma yoga is the recognition that all action belongs to the Supreme Being. When you have an inner attitude that all your actions come from God and belong to God, you are a Karma yogi. The inner dialogue of a Karma yogi is, "I am an instrument of the eternal infinite being. Every breath of mine, every act of mine is a divine movement of the infinite. My thoughts and actions come from the infinite and return to the infinite." True practice of Karma yoga leads to spontaneous detachment from outcome and one-pointed focused mindfulness as you perform your actions. Action from this level of consciousness is not binding; rather, it liberates you and enables you spontaneously to recognize that you are an eternal being on a cosmic journey. Karma yogis have no anxiety because they have no worry. The Karma yogi knows that God is performing the action and takes care of the results.

The fourth yoga is known as Raja yoga, the main subject of this book. Raja yoga is frequently referred to as the royal path to yoga because it is rich and abundant in knowledge and experience. Raja yoga can be practiced by anyone with a little bit of training.

Raja yoga is the path of union through practices that take your awareness inward. The essence of Raja yoga is an integration of body, mind, and soul through procedures that enhance mind-body coordination. These techniques awaken poise, grace, strength, and the development of centered awareness even in the midst of chaos and turmoil. They improve your physical health and your mental clarity while heightening your senses of perception. As a consequence of these practices, you are able to experience increased vitality along with better mental and physical capacity. Raja yogis have greater enjoyment of life, while enthusiasm and inspiration become an everyday experience.

Raja yoga helps you practice the other yogas with greater ease, effortlessness, and joy. When you feel physically vital, emotionally stable, and psychologically centered, your ability and desire to love and express authentic compassion expand. You become more capable of surrendering to the will of God and begin a never-ending journey of knowledge.

For those who feel that God is difficult to find, we want to encourage you to begin practicing the principles in this book. You will discover that God is not difficult to find. God is impossible to avoid, for there is nowhere that God is not.

Acknowledgments

This book is woven with the love of many beloved souls who share our journey.

We wish to thank our precious families, who lovingly support us in all the work we do: Rita, Mallika, Sumant and Tara, Gotham and Candice; Pam, Max, Sara, and Isabel.

To Ray Chambers, Jose Busquets, Charley Paz, and Howard Simon for their unwavering support of the Chopra Center mission.

To the John Wiley & Sons editorial team, Tom Miller and Kellam Ayres, for helping this book reach its full potential.

To the dedicated staff of the Chopra Center, who nurture every guest entering our place of healing and transformation: Bill Abasolo, Vicki Abrams, Leanne Backer, Catherine Baer, Paula Bass, Brent Becvar, Sanjeev Bhanot, Marina Bigo, Sandra Blazinski, Corrine Champigny, Janice Crawford, Nancy Ede, Kana Emidy-Mazza, Jenny Ephrom, Ana Fakhri, Ana Paula Fernandez, Patrick Fischer, Roger Gabriel, Lorri Gifford, David

Greenspan, Emily Hobgood, Gwyneth Hudson, Jennifer Johnson, Alisha Kaufman, Kenneth Kolonko, Totiana Lamberti, Joseph Lancaster, Justine Lawrence, Anastacia Leigh, Summer Lewis, Asha Maclsaac, Tufani Mayfield, Joelene Monestier, Bjorn Nagle, Kelly Peters-Luvera, Jessica Przygocki, Carolyn Rangel, Felicia Rangel, Kristy Reeves, Sharon Reif, Anna Rios, Jayme Rios, Teresa Robles, Julian Romero, Nicolas Ruiz, Stephanie Sanders, JoElla Shephard, Max Simon, Drew Tabatchnick, William Vargas, Katherine Weber, Dana Willoughby, Grace Wilson, and Kelly Worrall.

To Clair Diab for her leadership in the Seven Spiritual Laws of Yoga Teacher Training Program.

To Omry Reznick, Claire Diab, Michael Fukumura, Roger Gabriel, and Pam Simon for making the photos that saved us thousands of words.

To Geeta Singh for bringing the message around the world.

To Lynn Franklin for enabling this book to reach seekers of unity on every continent.

Introduction

*The source from which the world and the mind rise
and into which they set is termed Reality, which
does not rise nor does it subside.*

—Ramana Maharishi

I am not in the world; the world is in me." This daring declaration of ancient yogis gave expression to the perennial truth that the material universe, our physical bodies, and the thoughts that occupy our minds are expressions of an underlying unbounded field of consciousness. The "I" in the bold statement reflects a transformation in the internal reference of the seeker from skin-encapsulated ego to expanded spirit. These original explorers of consciousness charted a course for us to follow — the path of yoga. This is the path we follow.

We are deeply gratified by the expanding acceptance in the West of the philosophy and practices usually attributed to

I

the East. Through our books, lectures, and workshops, we have been sharing our understanding and experience of the Vedic and Yogic wisdom traditions because we believe that this knowledge has universal value. Just as no one would argue that gravity applies only to England because Sir Isaac Newton was British or that Einstein's theory of relativity was relevant only in Germany, we suggest that the profound insights gained through yoga are valuable for every person living on this planet, regardless of age, gender, or cultural inheritance. The principles of yoga are not limited by time or space.

As the human inhabitants of our world increasingly recognize themselves as members of a global village, ideas that were rejected by all but a few wild inner-space explorers thirty years ago are now resonating in our collective awareness. Just a few heartbeats back, the mention of yoga and meditation as essential components of a healthy lifestyle led to skepticism and even ridicule. But concepts that add genuine value to life eventually find their way into the light of human consciousness. Paraphrasing the great German philosopher, Arthur Schopenhauer, every great idea goes through three phases before it is accepted. In the first it is rejected, in the second it is ridiculed, and in the third it is held to be self-evident. The value that yoga brings to body, mind, and spirit is becoming increasingly obvious to a critical mass of people in North America and around the world.

Our relationship with yoga spans more than three decades. We learned early in our spiritual journey the value of alternating *asanas* (yoga poses), *pranayama* (breathing exercises), and meditation to stabilize aware-

ness while spending extended time in silence. In Seduc-
tion of Spirit, our intensive meditation course held twice
yearly at the Chopra Center, we repeatedly see the benefits that conscious movement brings to our guests, when
their attention is directed inward for hours each day. As a
result of our personal experience and that of thousands of
course participants, this book emerged.

The information and practices presented in this book
provide you with a path to expand your awareness of the
relationship between your individuality and your world.
Our planet is in need of healing and transformation.
With exploding population growth, the human footprint
on earth looms larger each day. People who understand
the relationship between individual and collective
choices cannot ignore the issues of social justice, eco-
nomic disparities, ecological disruption, and cultural
conflicts. At times, the challenges of our age can seem
overwhelming and beyond the influence of individual
intention. We believe, however, that each of us has an
opportunity to contribute to a better world through the
very personal choices we make on daily basis. Through the
Seven Spiritual Laws of Yoga program, you will enhance
the integration between your body and mind and develop
the practice of maintaining balance and flexibility in the
midst of challenge. You will gain increased access to your
creativity and intuition and become aware of how your
individual thoughts, words, and actions influence and are
influenced by your environment. As a result of this
awareness, you will contribute to the collective awakening
of world consciousness.

All of our work through the Chopra Center has been
based upon the core principle that consciousness is the

primary force in the universe. Consciousness gives rise to thought; thought gives rise to action. All change begins with awareness—awareness of the current situation, awareness of the potential for something greater, and awareness of the unlimited creativity that exists within each of us to catalyze the transformation we want to see for ourselves and for generations to follow.

Not long ago it seemed fanciful that public smoking would be restricted and tobacco companies would sponsor public service ads that discourage smoking, but this shift in awareness occurred when a critical mass of people decided they would no longer tolerate a behavior that harmed many while benefiting a few. In a similar way, we anticipate that as more people shift their inner attitude from What's in it for me? to How can I help? we will see an expanding sense of both individual and collective responsibility for the choices that are guiding the future of our planet. We are hopeful that as a result of the changes you experience through the practice of the Seven Spiritual Laws of Yoga program, you will be unable to resist the urge to contribute to the healing and transformation of humanity and the world.

The initial response to the Seven Spiritual Laws of Yoga program has been so enthusiastic that we have developed a yoga training program for those interested in bringing this knowledge and practice to their communities. From novices to experienced yoga teachers, people around the world are learning to teach others the principles and technology that enable them to apply the deep wisdom of yoga to daily life. If, after experiencing for yourself the transformational power of this program, you have the desire to share this knowledge with others, we welcome your participation. Together, we can remind the members of our global family that each of us has the ability to contribute to peace and harmony in the world by awakening these qualities within.

With love,
Deepak and David

PART I

The Philosophy of Yoga

1

Yoga Is Union

Without self-knowledge, we cannot go beyond the mind.

—*Jiddu Krishnamurti*

The proliferation of yoga classes and yoga centers throughout the Western world is a tribute to yoga's indisputable power to enliven physical well-being. In cities across North America, Europe, and Australia, yoga studios offer students a vast range of styles and techniques designed to enhance fitness. Yoga postures can increase your flexibility, strengthen your muscles, improve your posture, and enhance your circulation. Athletic programs from gymnastics to football now incorporate yoga for its systematic approach to stretching muscles, tendons, and joints. Fitness enthusiasts are often pleasantly surprised by how quickly the addition of yoga postures to a workout routine can improve tone and posture.

If the practice of yoga provided only these physical benefits, it would fully justify its place in our lives. However, at its core, yoga is much more than a system of physical fitness. It is a science of balanced living, a path for realizing full human potential. In these tumultuous times, yoga provides an anchor to a quieter domain of life, enabling people living in a modern technological world to stay connected to their natural humanity. Yoga offers the promise of remaining centered in the midst of turbulence.

The essential purpose of yoga is the integration of all the layers of life—environmental, physical, emotional, psychological, and spiritual. The word *yoga* is derived from the Sanskrit root *yuj*, which means "to unite." It is related to the English word *yoke*. A farmer yoking two oxen to pull his plow is performing an action that hints at the essence of a spiritual experience. At its core, yoga means union, the union of body, mind, and soul; the union of the ego and the spirit; the union of the mundane and the divine.

The Seven Spiritual Laws in Action

The Seven Spiritual Laws of Yoga program will raise your level of physical vitality, clear emotional blockages from your heart, and awaken your joyfulness and enthusiasm for life. Since its release in 1994, Deepak's book *The Seven Spiritual Laws of Success* has improved the lives of millions of readers around the world. Through seven easily understood principles, *The Seven Spiritual Laws of Success* proclaims that harmony, happiness, and abundance are available to anyone willing to embrace a consciousness-based approach to life. Our yoga program brings the seven laws into action through the principles and techniques of a consciousness-based practice.

We celebrate the rising popularity of yoga in the Western world. Even if your primary motivation for taking a yoga class is to lose weight or to develop a more muscular body, you cannot escape the subtler benefits of enhanced vitality and a noticeable reduction in your stress level. Yoga is a practical system to awaken human potential. It does not require you to believe in a set of principles in order to reap its benefits. On the contrary, the regular practice of yoga naturally generates a healthy belief system based upon your direct experience of the world through a more flexible nervous system. Perform yoga poses on a regular basis and your mind and emotions will change.

Yoga is a central component of the comprehensive system of Indian philosophy known as Vedic science. With roots in the Indus Valley civilization going back over five thousand years, the Vedas represent the poetic cognitions of enlightened sages on the origins of the universe and the evolution of life. The English word *wisdom* traces its origins to the primitive Germanic word *wid*, meaning "to know." *Wid*, in turn, is derived from the Sanskrit word *Veda*, meaning "external knowledge." The Vedas are the expression of perennial wisdom, and yoga is the practical aspect of Vedic science. Yoga is a system through which human beings can directly access the wisdom of life. Practitioners of yoga—*yogis*—are dynamic and creative forces for positive change. A yogi knows that his mind and body are in the ever-changing world, but his essence—his soul—resides in a dimension that is beyond change.

The Seven Spiritual Laws of Yoga program is designed for those who wish to take their yoga practice to a deeper level, using their bodies to access more expanded levels of their minds. This is the time-honored value of yoga—to cultivate an inner state of centered awareness that cannot be disturbed by the inevitable turmoil of life.

Layers of Life

People are complex and multifaceted beings with many rich layers, although the Western scientific model of a person tends to reflect the Newtonian mechanistic view of life that sees people as primarily physical entities—biological machines that have learned to think. Despite the fact that almost a century ago the discoveries of quantum physics revealed that the material model of life is incomplete, modern medicine and physiology continue to view people as primarily composed of molecules.

According to this predominantly physical perspective, if you are feeling depressed, it is not because you are harboring anger and resentment over the affair your spouse had with your best friend; rather, it is the result of inadequate levels of serotonin in your brain. If you simply enhance the level of this neurotransmitter molecule through the appropriate selective serotonin reuptake inhibitor, your depression will vanish. If your blood pressure is elevated, it is not the consequence of constant strain with your demanding boss; rather, it is the result of excessive levels of the chemical angiotensin. Take an angiotensin converting enzyme inhibitor and your blood pressure will normalize. If you have trouble sleeping at night, your excessive credit card debt is not to blame; your brain is simply not producing sufficient concentrations of gamma-aminobutyric acid. Any of a number of medications will correct this deficiency and you will sleep as soundly as a baby.

This material approach can be remarkably effective in the short-term relief of symptoms. Unfortunately, it rarely promotes a deeper understanding of life, it rarely leads to healing and transformation, and the side effects of medications are often limiting.

Expanding the vision of life beyond a purely bio-chemical perspective, yoga reminds us that we live life simultaneously on many levels. The essence of yoga is to find the unity in the diversity of our multidimensionality. Throughout the centuries, great yoga teachers have awakened their contemporaries to the fascinating paradox that although to the mind and senses the world is an ever-changing experience, from the perspective of spirit, the infinite diversity of forms and phenomena is simply the disguise of an underlying nonchanging reality.

Adi Shankara, the Sage of Sages

One of the most influential teachers of the philosophy of yoga and Veda was the ninth-century sage Adi Shankara. Known as the greatest revivalist of Vedic science, he elegantly elaborated the layers of life that mask the essential spiritual self. Born in A.D. 805, Shankara is said to have been fluent in Sanskrit by the age of one and to have mastered all sacred literature by age eight. He began writing his own commentaries on the Vedas by age fifteen and was recognized as the leading authority on yoga by the time he turned twenty. He established seats of learning throughout India with one goal in mind—to help human beings overcome their suffering through the wisdom of life. His approach to truth was called *Advaita,* meaning "nondualism." The essence of Shankara's teaching is that one underlying field of intelligence manifests as the multiplicity of forms and phenomena that we call the physical universe.

It is helpful to recognize the disguises consciousness dons so you can see through to the underlying reality. This is the great game of hide-and-seek that spirit plays with us. The nonlocal field of awareness gives rise to the sensory world that overshadows our experience of the underlying unity. At some point we recognize that the world of sensations alone cannot bring us genuine peace or happiness, so we begin our journey of uncovering the layers that mask our essential unbounded nature. Shankara called these various layers *koshas,* meaning "coverings," and he categorized them into three primary divisions—a physical body, a subtle body, and a causal body. We can also say body, mind, and soul. Let's explore each of these primary divisions and their three secondary layers.

The Physical Body— The Field of Molecules

Within your physical domain, you have an extended body, a personal body, and an energetic body. Your extended body is the environment, containing the never-

The Layers of Life

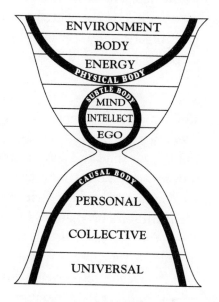

ENVIRONMENT
BODY
ENERGY
PHYSICAL BODY
SUBTLE BODY
MIND
INTELLECT
EGO
CAUSAL BODY
PERSONAL
COLLECTIVE
UNIVERSAL

ending supply of energy and information that is available to you. Every sound, sensation, sight, flavor, and aroma you ingest from the environment influences your body and mind. Although your senses may tell you otherwise, there is no distinct boundary between your personal and extended bodies, which are in constant and dynamic exchange. Each breath that you inhale and exhale is a reminder of the continuous conversation taking place between your physical body and your environment.

This recognition requires you to take responsibility for what is happening in your environment. As a yogi, you are an environmentalist because you recognize that the rivers flowing through the valleys and those flowing through your veins are intimately related. The breath of an old-growth forest and your most recent breath are inextricably intertwined. The quality of the soil in which your food is raised is directly connected to the health of your tissues and organs. Your environment is your extended body. You are inseparably interwoven with your ecosystem.

Of course, you do have a personal body that consists of the molecules that temporarily comprise your cells, tissues, and organs. We say temporarily because although it appears that your body is solid and constant, it actually is continuously transforming. Scientific studies using radio-isotope tracings convincingly show that 98 percent of the ten trillion quadrillion (10^{28}) atoms in your body are replaced annually. Your stomach lining re-creates itself about every five days, your skin is made anew every month, and your liver cells turn over every six weeks. Although your body appears to be fixed and stable, it is continually metamorphosing.

The vast majority of the cells in your body are derived from the food you eat. Recognizing this, Shankara named the physical body *annamaya kosha*, meaning "the covering made of food." To create and maintain a healthy body, yogis pay attention to the food they consume, minimizing the toxicity they ingest while maximizing the nourishment they receive. Certain foods are said to be particularly conducive to a yogic lifestyle. These foods are known as *sattvic*, which means they contribute to the purity of the body. The four most sattvic foods revered by yogis are almonds, honey, milk, and ghee (clarified butter). Getting a daily dose of these foods benefits the body, mind, and soul of a person dedicated to creating greater mind-body integration. When acknowledging the relationship between your personal and extended bodies be certain to consume only organic dairy products.

Shankara called the third layer of the physical body *pranamaya kosha,* meaning "the sheath made of vital energy." There is a difference between the cells of a corpse and the cells of a vibrant living being. This organizing principle that breathes life into biochemicals is called *prana.* There are five seats of prana in the body, localized in the head, throat, heart, stomach, and pelvis. These centers of movement govern the flow of life force throughout the body. When prana is moving freely throughout the cells and tissues, vitality and creativity are abundant. Yogic breathing exercises, known as *pranayama* techniques, are designed to awaken and purify the vital energy layer of the body. We'll be exploring these powerful approaches in chapter 4.

The Subtle Body—The Mind Field

Most people identify themselves with their mind, intellect, and ego, which are the components of the subtle body. The seventeenth-century French philosopher René Descartes is famous for his statement, *"Cogito, ergo sum,"* meaning "I think, therefore I am." People continue to believe that they are their minds, but Shankara encourages us to recognize that the components of our subtle body are simply coverings of the soul.

According to this framework, the mind is the repository of sensory impressions. When you hear a sound, feel a sensation, see a sight, taste a flavor, or smell a fragrance, the sensory experience registers in your consciousness at a level of your being called *manomaya kosha*. The mind cycles through different states of consciousness, and your sensory experiences change with these changing states. The impressions that enter your awareness during a waking state are different from those generated during dreaming. Yoga reminds us that reality is different in different states of consciousness—different filters of the mind layer.

The second layer of the subtle body is the intellect, known as *buddhimaya kosha*. This is the aspect of mind that discriminates. Whether you are trying to decide what kind of toothpaste to purchase, which partner to choose, or what house to buy, your intellect is at work, attempting to calculate the advantages and disadvantages of every choice you make. This layer integrates information based upon your beliefs and feelings to come to a decision. According to yoga, the ultimate purpose of this intellectual layer is to distinguish the real from the unreal. The real is that which cannot be lost whereas the unreal is anything that has a beginning and end to it. Knowing the difference is the essence of yoga.

The third layer of the subtle body is the ego. The ego is known in yoga as *ahankara*, which means the "I-former." According to Shankara, the ego is that aspect of your being that identifies with the positions and possessions of your life. It is ultimately your self-image—the way you want to project who you are to yourself and to the world.

The ego is the boundary maker that attempts to assert ownership through the concepts of "I," "me," "my," and "mine." The ego seeks security through control and often has a deep-seated need for approval. Most emotional pain is the result of your ego being offended because

Yoga Is Union   19

something that it believed it had control over was actually outside your jurisdiction.

It is easy to become lost in the subtle body, with its attachments to roles, relationships, and objects, but Shankara encourages us to go deeper. Letting go of the body and letting go of the mind open the possibility of experiencing an aspect of your being that is beyond your usual limitations. This is the realm of spirit, which Shankara called the causal body.

The Causal Body—The Field of Pure Potentiality

According to yoga, underlying the field of molecules we call the physical body and the field of thoughts called the subtle body is a realm of life known as the causal body or the domain of spirit. Although we cannot perceive or measure this sphere of life, it gives rise to our thoughts, feelings, dreams, desires, and memories, as well as to the molecules that make up our bodies and the material world. Like the physical body and the subtle body, the causal body has three layers.

The *personal* domain of spirit is the layer where the seeds of memories and desires are sown. According to Shankara, each person arrives on this planet with a specific purpose and a unique set of talents. Given the right environment, the seeds sprout, and you become capable of expressing your gifts in the world. Although the modern material model of life suggests that their genes determine people's talents, we only have to look at identical twins to realize that the same molecular structure does not determine an individual's nature. Pregnant mothers report that even in the womb, different babies express different tendencies.

According to Shankara, every individual has a personal soul with its unique memories and desires. These memories and desires guide the course of your life. When you nurture the seeds of your innate gifts with your attention and intention, they sprout, and your personal soul finds fulfillment.

The second sheath of the causal body is the *collective domain*. This realm impels you to live a life of mythic proportions. The gods and goddesses that reside in the collective domain within your soul have one desire—to express their creative power through you. Each of us is on a heroic journey in search of the Holy Grail. Along the way, obstacles and challenges arise, forcing us to reach deeper into our being.

These collective aspirations are translated into the archetypal stories that people have been telling one another for millennia. For example, we learn the risks associated with the arrogance of power through the tragic story of Icarus. Ignoring the advice of his father, he flew too close to the sun, melted his waxen wings, and crashed into the ocean. If Bill Clinton or Martha Stewart had heeded the wisdom resonating in their collective domain, they might have avoided their foretold painful outcomes.

A woman who closes down when a relationship becomes too intimate is living the myth of Daphne who, overwhelmed by the pursuit of Apollo, is transformed into a laurel tree. A young man seeking to reestablish a formerly successful family business is reenacting the story of Jason and the Argonauts. The stories unfolding in our lives and those around us are perennial stories.

The mythic gods and goddesses are alive and well within our collective domain. We can see the expression of Queen Juno in the powerful women of our era—Margaret Thatcher, Golda Meir, Hillary Clinton. The goddess of nature, Diana, shows her modern face through Jane Goodall and Julia "Butterfly" Hill. Venus made her most direct appearance via Marilyn Monroe, while Dionysus, the god of intoxication and excess, has a tendency to show up in the stream of people who require stays at the Betty Ford Clinic.

You are a living story. Become aware of the stories you tell about yourself and your world. Participate consciously in the writing of the next chapter of your life. Yoga encourages you to expand your sense of self to embrace the collective domain of your soul. This is where the deepest aspirations of humanity find fulfillment through the perennial stories we tell ourselves and our children.

According to Shankara, the deepest aspect of your being is beyond time, space, and causality, yet gives rise to the manifest universe. This is the *universal* domain of spirit in which all distinctions merge in unity. Having no qualities of its own, this field of pure potentiality manifests as the infinitely diverse world of forms and phenomena. The unbounded ocean of being disguises itself in the sheaths of the causal, subtle, and physical realms.

This nonlocal, unbounded realm is the source and goal of life. Yoga encourages us to bring our attention to this universal domain so that we become imbued with the deep stillness and creativity it represents. Then, even as we are engaged in dynamic activity, we retain the silence and centered awareness of universal spirit.

The vision of life as elaborated by Shankara is as useful today as it was centuries ago. For seekers of greater well-being, vitality, and wisdom, Shankara offers a map that ultimately leads to the soul.

The Seven Spiritual Laws of Yoga program provides the technology to support this journey. Whether you are new to yoga or have been practicing for some time, we intend for this program to shift your awareness. Marcel Proust wrote, "The real journey of discovery is not in seeking new landscapes, but in seeing with new eyes." It is our intention that the Seven Spiritual Laws of Yoga program will enable you to see your environment, body, mind, and emotions from a new perspective.

This subtle shift in consciousness can be a powerful catalytic force for healing and transformation in your life. Try this program for a month, and you will see changes, not only in your practice of poses but also in your life as a whole.

2

Soul Questions

Nothing here below is profane for those who know how to see. On the contrary, everything is sacred.
—Pierre Teilhard de Chardin

The generally recognized founder of yoga philosophy is the legendary sage Maharishi Patanjali, whose life is shrouded in the mists of myth and history. According to one story, his mother, Gonnika, was praying for a child to Lord Vishnu, the god who maintains the universe. Vishnu was so moved by her purity and devotion that he asked his beloved cosmic serpent, Ananta, to prepare for human incarnation. A tiny speck of Ananta's celestial body fell into Gonnika's upturned palms. She nurtured this cosmic seed with her love until it developed into a baby boy. She named her child Patanjali from the word *pat*, meaning "descended from heaven," and *anjali*, the word for her praying posture. This being, whose life historians date back two centuries before the birth of Christ, elaborated the principles of yoga for the benefit of humanity.

In his classic work, the *Yoga Sutras*, Patanjali sets the goal of yoga as nothing short of total freedom from suffering. To fulfill this worthy intention, Patanjali elaborated the eight branches of yoga. Each of these components of yoga helps you shift your internal reference point from constricted to expanded consciousness. As you move from local to nonlocal awareness, your internal reference point spontaneously transforms from ego to spirit, which enables you to see the bigger picture when facing any challenge.

According to Patanjali, whenever we are solely identified with our ego, we bind ourselves to things that do not have permanent reality. This may be attachment to a relationship, a job, a body, or a material possession. It may be attachment to a belief or an idea of the way things should be. Whatever the object of attachment is, the binding of your identity to something that resides in the world of forms and phenomena is the seed cause of distress, unhappiness, and illness. Remembering that the real you is not trapped in the volume of a body for the span of a lifetime is the key to genuine freedom and joy. Yoga is designed to give you a glimpse of your essential self by taking you from deep silence into dynamic action and back again to profound stillness. In the practice of the Seven Spiritual Laws of Yoga program, you will experience this full range of yoga—stillness to activity and back to stillness.

. . .

Yoga philosophy begins with the spirit. Getting in touch with your spirit is the true goal of yoga. It occurs naturally when your mind quiets and you are able to access the inner wisdom that emerges from the deepest aspect of your being. One way to connect with your soul is by consciously asking yourself questions that go to the heart of the human experience. There are three key questions that help shift your internal reference point from ego to spirit. They are:

Who am I?
What do I want?
How can I serve?

Whether or not you are aware of it, these questions are directing your choices in life. Regularly bringing your current answers to conscious awareness enables you to be alert to the opportunities that resonate with the needs of your soul.

When asked the question, Who are you? most people usually identify themselves in terms of their positions and possessions. You might say, "I am the chief financial officer of a software company," or "I am a high school math teacher." You may identify with where you live, saying, "I am a New Yorker," or "I'm Canadian." You may identify yourself in terms of a relationship by responding, "I am the assistant to the president," or "I am a mother." Although we all have the tendency to identify ourselves with roles, objects, and relationships in our lives, yoga encourages us to go deeper into our being and find the inner place that is beyond external anchors. This is the source of all energy and creativity in life. When you begin to recognize that your essential nature is unbounded and eternal, life becomes joyful, meaningful, and carefree.

Try this simple exercise to become aware of your current internal reference point. Simply close your eyes, take a few slow, deep breaths, and settle your awareness in the area of your heart. Now silently ask yourself the question, Who am I? every fifteen seconds. Listen innocently to the answers that emerge from your deeper mind.

As you perform this process, you may recognize that you define yourself by the roles you play, answering the question, Who am I? with:

I am . . .
a computer programmer
the vice president of marketing
a pediatric nurse

You may define yourself by a group with which you identify.

I am . . .
an American
a New York Yankees fan
a Libertarian

You may define yourself in terms of a relationship.

I am . . .
a single parent
a loving spouse
a devoted daughter

You may see yourself in terms of certain practices you perform.

I am . . .
a vegetarian
a triathlete
a meditator

From the perspective of yoga, each of these identity points represents some aspect of you but not the ultimate essence of who you are. Asking the second question of the soul, What do I want? takes you deeper. In the Upanishads, one of the crown jewels in the Vedic body of literature, there is the expression, "You are what your deep, driving desire is. As is your desire, so is your will. As is your will, so is your deed. As is your deed, so is your destiny." When you know what a person desires, you know the essence of that person. To become more aware of your deep desires, close your eyes and ask yourself every fifteen seconds the questions:

What do I want?
What do I really want?

Different levels of your being give rise to different desires. Your physical body has intrinsic needs for food, water, oxygen, and sexual gratification. Listening to the desires of your body and providing nourishing fulfillment ensure health and vitality. Your subtle body has needs for emotional connection, achievement, and recognition. Expressing your talents and honoring the contributions made by others ensure the health and well-being of your subtle body. Your causal body has the need for creative expression and renewal. It has the need for unity to predominate over diversity, for expansiveness over restriction.

The spiritual journey is one of fulfilling the needs of the flesh, the needs of the mind, and the needs of the spirit. When you are willing to pose the question to yourself, What do I really want? you are asking what level of your being is expressing a need. Listen to the answers that arise from within you and write them down. Watch how over time your desires become fulfilled or are transformed in different expressions. Whether they are satisfied or change, new desires will arise to fill the void. Become conscious of the forces that drive your choices and you will become more intimate with your essential nature. This will deepen your connection to your soul, which is the goal of yoga.

As you become increasingly conscious of your identity and your desires, ask yourself the third soul question, How can I serve? Again, close your eyes, bring your attention into the area of your heart, and ask yourself these questions, listening to the responses that emerge from a deeper aspect of your being:

How can I serve?
How can I be of service?
How can I help?
How can I best serve?

The inner dialogue of the subtle body revolves around the questions, What do I get out of this? What's in it for me? As your inner reference point expands to embrace your causal body, your inner dialogue shifts to, How can I help? As your sense of self expands, your compassion proportionately increases and you naturally find yourself caring about how your choices influence those around you.

Yogic sages would agree that the first-century Rabbi Hillel's questions are worth asking:

If I am not for myself, who will be for me?
If I am only for myself, what am I?
If not now, when?

The true purpose of yoga is to discover that aspect of your being that can never be lost. Your job may change, your relationships may change, your body may change, your beliefs may change, your desires may change, your ideas about your role in the world may change, but the essence of who you are is the continuity of awareness that has no beginning or end. Your thoughts, beliefs, expectations, goals, and experiences may come and go, but the one who is having the experiences—the experiencer—remains.

As you progress in your practice, you may find that the answers to the questions, Who am I? What do I want? and How can I serve? emerge from a deeper layer of your being. You may find your sense of identity changing, reflecting a more expanded view of your self. You may find your desires becoming less personal. As your concept of self expands, your concern about others may simultaneously increase. You may discover a deepening aspiration to make a contribution to your community and your world. This expansion of self-awareness is the essence of yoga.

3

The Royal Path
to Union

*In the attitude of silence the soul finds the path in a
clearer light, and what is elusive and deceptive
resolves itself into crystal clearness.*
                                        —Mahatma Gandhi

Your body is a field of molecules. Your mind is a field of
thoughts. Underlying and giving rise to your body
and your mind is a field of consciousness—the domain of
spirit. To know yourself as an unbounded spirit disguised as
a body/mind frees you to live with confidence and compassion, with love and enthusiasm. To remove the veils
that hide the deepest layers of your being, Maharishi
Patanjali elaborated the eight branches of yoga—*Yama,
Niyama, Asana, Pranayama, Pratyahara, Dharana, Dhyana,*
and *Samadhi.* They are sometimes referred to as the eight

limbs (*asthanga*) of yoga, but they are not to be seen as sequential stages. Rather, they serve as different entry points into an expanded sense of self through interpretations, choices, and experiences that remind you of your essential nature. These are the components of *Raja yoga*, the royal path to union. Let's review each of them in some detail.

The First Branch of Yoga—Yama

Yama is most commonly translated as the "rules of social behavior." They are the universal guidelines for engaging with others. The Yamas are traditionally described as

1. practicing nonviolence
2. speaking truthfully
3. exercising appropriate sexual control
4. being honest
5. being generous

All spiritual and religious traditions encourage people to live ethical lives. Yoga agrees but concedes that living a life in perfect harmony with your environment is difficult from the level of morality—through a prescribed set of shoulds and should-nots. Patanjali describes the yamas as the spontaneously evolutionary behavior of an enlightened being.

If you recognize that your individuality is intimately woven into the fabric of life—that you are a strand in the web of life—you lose the ability to act in ways that are harmful to yourself or others. You adhere to the rules of social conduct because you are behaving from the level of spontaneous right action. This state of behaving in accordance with natural law is called *Kriya Shakti*. Although the Sanskrit words *kriya* and *karma* both mean "action," kriya is action that does not generate reaction, as opposed to karma, which automatically generates proportionate consequences. There are no personal consequences when you are acting from the level of Kriya Shakti because you do not generate any resistance. People sometimes describe this state as being "in the flow" or "in the zone."

Acting from this level of your soul, you are incapable of being violent because your whole being is established in peace. This is the essence of the first Yama, known in Sanskrit as *ahimsa*. Your thoughts are nonviolent, your words are nonviolent, and your actions are nonviolent. Violence cannot arise because your heart and mind are filled with love and compassion for the human condition. Mahatma Gandhi championed the principle of nonviolence in the independence movement of India from Britain. He said, "If you express your love in such a manner that it impresses itself indelibly upon your so-called enemy, he must return that love . . . and that requires far greater courage than delivering of blows."

The second Yama is truthfulness, or *satya*. Truthfulness derives from a state of being in which you are able to distinguish your observations from your interpretations. You accept the world as it is, recognizing that reality is a selective act of attention and interpretation. Recognizing that truth is different for different people, you commit to life-supporting choices that are aligned with an expanded view of self. Patanjali described truth as the integrity of thought, word, and action. You speak the sweet truth and are inherently honest because truthfulness is an expression of your commitment to a spiritual life. The short-term benefits of distorting the truth are outweighed by the discomfort that arises from betraying your integrity. Ultimately you recognize truth, love, and God to be different expressions of the same undifferentiated reality.

Brahmacharya, the third Yama, is often translated as "celibacy." We believe this is a limited view of this yama. The word is derived from *achara*, meaning "pathway," and *brahman*, meaning "unity consciousness." In Vedic society, people traditionally chose one of two paths to enlightenment—the path of the householder and the path of a renunciate. For those choosing the path of a monk or a nun, the path to unity consciousness naturally includes forsaking sexual activity. For the vast majority of people choosing the householder path, brahmacharya means rejoicing in the healthy expression of sexual energy. One interpretation of the word *charya* is "grazing," suggesting that brahmacharya connotes partaking of the sacred as you are engaged in your daily life.

The essential creative power of the universe is sexual, and you are a loving manifestation of that energy. Seeing the entire creation as an expression of the divine impulse to generate, you celebrate the creative forces. Brahmacharya means aligning with the creative energy of the cosmos. Ultimately, as your soul makes love with the cosmos, your need to express your sexuality may be supplanted by a more expanded expression of love.

The fourth Yama, *asteya*, or honesty, means relinquishing the idea that things outside yourself will provide you security and happiness. Asteya is being established in a state of nongrasping. Lack of honesty almost always derives from fear of loss—loss of money, love, position, power. The ability to live an honest life is based upon a deep connection to spirit. When inner fullness predominates, you lose the need to manipulate, obscure, or deceive. Honesty is the intrinsic state of a person living a life of integrity. According to yoga, life-supporting, evolutionary behaviors are the natural consequence of expanded awareness.

The fifth Yama, generosity, or *aparigraha*, derives from the shift in internal reference from predominantly ego-based to predominantly spirit-based. A yogi who knows that his essential nature is nonlocal spontaneously expresses generosity in every thought, word, and action. Constricted awareness reinforces limitations. Expanded awareness generates abundance consciousness. This Yama implies the absence of aversion. Established in aparigraha, your attachment to the accumulation of material possessions loses its hold on you. It doesn't mean you don't enjoy the world; you are simply not imprisoned by it. The practice of yoga, which cultivates expanded awareness, awakens generosity because nature is generous.

The Second Branch of Yoga—Niyama

The second limb of yoga as outlined by Patanjali is *Niyama*, traditionally interpreted as the "rules of personal behavior." We see them as the qualities naturally expressed in an evolutionary personality. How do you live when no one is looking? What choices do you make when you are the only witness? The Niyamas of yoga encourage

1. purity

2. contentment

3. discipline

4. spiritual exploration

5. surrender to the divine

Again, these qualities do not arise by making a mood of moral self-righteousness, but they emerge as a result of a person living a natural, balanced life. H. G. Wells said, "Moral indignation is jealousy with a halo," and yoga would agree.

Like ideal social conduct, evolutionary personal qualities derive from your connection to spirit. Focusing on the first Niyama, purity, or *shoucha*, adds no value to life if it encourages a judgmental mind-set, but it is of great value if you see your choices in terms of nourishment versus toxicity. Your body and mind are constructed from the impressions that you ingest from the environment. The sounds, sensations, sights, tastes, and smells carry the energy and information that are metabolized into you. Yoga encourages you to consciously choose experiences that are nourishing to your body, mind, and soul.

Contentment, or *santosha*, the second Niyama, is the fragrance of present moment awareness. When you struggle against the present moment, you struggle against the entire cosmos. Contentment, however, does not imply acquiescence. Yogis are committed in thought, word, and deed to supporting evolutionary change that enhances the well-being of all sentient creatures on this planet. Contentment implies acceptance without resignation.

Contentment emerges when you relinquish your

attachment to the need for control, power, and approval. Santosha is the absence of addiction to power, sensation, and security. Through the practice of yoga, your experience of the present moment quiets the mental turbulence that disturbs your contentment—contentment that reflects a state of being in which your peace is independent of situations and circumstances happening around you.

The third Niyama, *tapas*, is traditionally translated as "discipline" or "austerity." The word *tapas* means "fire." When the fire of a yogi's life is burning brightly, she is a beacon of light radiating balance and peace to the world. The fire is also responsible for digesting both nourishment and toxicity. A healthy inner fire can metabolize all impurities.

People often associate discipline with deprivation. The lives of people established in a yogic lifestyle may appear to be disciplined because their biological rhythms are aligned with the rhythms of nature. They arise early, meditate daily, exercise regularly, eat in a healthful and balanced way, and go to bed early because they directly experience the benefits of harmonizing their personal rhythms with those of nature. Tapas is embracing transformation as the pathway to higher consciousness.

Self-study, or *svadhyana*, is the fourth Niyama. Traditionally, this is interpreted as being dedicated to the study of spiritual literature, but at its heart, self-study means looking inside. There is a difference between knowledge and knowingness. Yoga advises us not to confuse information with wisdom, and self-study helps you understand the distinction. Self-study encourages self-referral as opposed to object referral. Your value and security come from a deep connection to spirit rather than from the things with which you are surrounded. When svadhyana is lively in your awareness, joy arises from within rather than being dependent upon outer accomplishments or acquisitions.

The final Niyama, *Ishwara-Pranidhana*, is often translated as "faith" or "surrendering to God." Ishwara is the personalized aspect of the infinite. Even when considering the boundless, the human mind wants to create boundaries. Ishwara is the name applied that makes familiar the infinite and unbounded field of intelligence. Ultimately, Ishwara-Pranidhana is surrendering to the wisdom of uncertainty. The seeds of wisdom are sown when you surrender to the unknown. The known is the past. True transformation, healing, and creativity flow out of present moment awareness, which means relinquishing your attachment to the past and embracing uncertainty.

A deeply spiritual friend of ours once contacted us from the coronary care unit at a New York hospital to say he had just had an emergency three-vessel coronary artery bypass operation. Only forty-two years old, he had never smoked, he was a vegetarian, and he meditated regularly. We obviously were very concerned about how he was doing and feeling, but he quickly reassured us he was doing well and was confident that everything would work out fine.

He explained that a few days earlier he had been visiting Long Island and had driven to Coney Island to ride on the roller coasters. He enjoyed riding the roller coasters because despite the turbulence, he knew he was safe. In an analogous way, because of his deep connection to spirit, our friend was able to surrender to the unknown when a blood vessel to his heart suddenly became blocked. He trusted that despite the twists and turns his life was taking, he would be okay whatever the outcome. This is Ishwara-Pranidhana—surrender to the divine.

The Yamas and Niyamas represent the inner dialogue of a yogi. These are not qualities one can make a mood of or manipulate. They arise spontaneously as the natural expression of a more expanded sense of self. You can see them as milestones of your spiritual progress. Allow them to resonate in your awareness, avoiding the impulse to be self-critical or judgmental when you occasionally fail to express the highest value of each principle. To awaken spontaneous evolutionary thought and action in your being, Patanjali encourages you to put your attention on more refined aspects of your body, your breath, your senses, and your mind. These are the next branches of yoga.

The Third Branch of Yoga—Asana

The word *asana* means "seat" or "position." When people consider yoga, they usually think of this branch, which refers to the postures people enter into to achieve physical flexibility and tone. At a deeper level, asana means the full expression of mind-body integration, in which you become consciously aware of the flow of life energy in your body. Performing asanas with full awareness is practice for performing action in life with awareness.

In the great Indian epic, the *Bhagavad Gita*, Lord Krishna instructs the archetypal human Arjuna first to become established in being, then to perform action in accordance with evolutionary law. The expression in Sanskrit is "Yogastah kurukarmani," which means "Established in yoga, perform action." *Yoga* here refers to the unified, integrated state of body, mind, and spirit.

The postures of yoga offer tremendous benefit to your body and mind. They help create balance, flexibility, and strength—all essential qualities for a healthy, dynamic life. When performed vigorously in sets, yoga can also be a powerful aerobic exercise to improve your cardiovascular fitness.

In addition to the direct benefits during the performance of postures, asanas provide enduring value throughout the day. If you perform asanas regularly, you will feel more flexible physically and emotionally. Flexibility is the essential difference between the vitality of youth and the lassitude of old age. Here is a yogic expression that we find inspiring: "Infinite flexibility is the secret to immortality." Like a palm tree that adapts to rather than resists gale force winds, a flexible body and mind enable you to adapt to the inevitable changes that life offers. Regular practice of yoga asanas cultivates flexibility while helping to release stagnating toxins from your body that inhibit the free flow of vital energy.

In the Seven Spiritual Laws of Yoga program, we have chosen asanas that enhance the flexibility of your joints, improve your balance, strengthen your muscles, and calm your mind. If you combine flexibility, balance, strength, and inner peace, you can surmount any obstacle. We will explore in great detail the most important yoga positions in chapter 5.

The Fourth Branch of Yoga— Pranayama

Prana is life force. It is the essential energy that animates inert matter into living, evolving biological beings. As first-year medical students, we took classes in gross anatomy in which there was the implied assumption that studying a cadaver could teach us about life. At the turn of the twentieth century, scientists would weigh someone immediately before and after they died to see if they could quantify what had left. (They did not record a difference, concluding that the soul did not weigh anything.)

From the perspective of yoga, the difference between a living being and a cadaver is the presence of prana, or vital energy.

When prana is flowing freely throughout your body/mind, you will feel healthy and vibrant. When prana is blocked, fatigue and disease soon follow. The concept of an animating force is present in every major wisdom and healing tradition. It is known as *chi* or *qi* in Traditional Chinese Medicine and *ruach* in the Kabalistic tradition. According to Patanjali, a key way to enliven prana is through conscious breathing techniques known as *pranayama*.

Pranayama means mastering the life force. There is an intimate relationship between your breath and your mind. When your mind is centered and quiet, so is your breath. When your mind is turbulent, your breathing becomes disordered. There are a number of classic pranayama breathing exercises that we will show you in chapter

4 that are designed to cleanse, balance, and invigorate the body. Just as your breath is affected by your mental activity, your mind can be influenced by conscious regulation of your breathing. Pranayama is a powerful technology to enhance neurorespiratory integration.

Prana is the life force that flows throughout nature and the universe. When you are tuned into the pranic energy in your body, you spontaneously become more attuned to the relationship between your individuality and your universality. In this way, pranayama can take you from a constricted state to an expanded state of awareness.

The Fifth Branch of Yoga— Pratyahara

Patanjali encourages us to take time withdrawing our senses from the world to hear our inner voice more clearly. *Pratyahara* is the process of directing the senses inward to become aware of the subtle elements of sound, touch, sight, taste, and smell. Ultimately all experience is in consciousness. When you look at a flower in your garden, your eyes receive frequencies of electromagnetic radiation that trigger chemical reactions in the rods and cones at the back of your eyes. As a result of these chemical changes in your retinas, electrical impulses are generated that eventually reach the visual cortex at the back of your brain. The interpretation of these fluctuations in energy and information takes place in your consciousness.

Although you imagine that you are seeing the flower outside of you, you are actually experiencing it within you on the screen of your awareness. This is why the great yogis say, "I am not in the world; the world is in me."

Pratyahara is the process of tuning into your subtle sensory experiences known in yoga as the *tanmatras*. Within your awareness are the seeds of sound, sensation, sight, taste, and scent. By going inside yourself, you can access these impulses and directly experience the knowledge that the world of forms and phenomena is a projection of your awareness.

You can awaken the tanmatras by consciously activating subtle sensory impressions on the screen of your awareness. Ask a friend to read these descriptions to you while your eyes are closed.

SOUND

Imagine . . .
the ringing of a church bell
the buzzing of a mosquito in your ear
the roar of an ocean wave crashing
against the shore

TOUCH

Imagine . . .
the feel of a fine cashmere sweater
the softness of a baby's skin
drops of rain falling on your face during
a summer shower

SIGHT

Imagine . . .
a sunset over a calm ocean
a fireworks display
the face of your mother

TASTE

Imagine . . .
biting into a luscious fresh strawberry
a spoonful of rich chocolate ice cream
a pungent jalapeno pepper

SMELL

Imagine . . .
the smell of the rich earth after a spring rain
the fragrance of blooming lilacs
the aroma of a bakery

Pratyahara is the process of temporarily withdrawing the senses from the outer world in order to recognize the sensations of your inner world. In a way, Pratyahara can be seen as sensory fasting. The word is comprised of *prati*, meaning "away," and *ahara*, meaning "food." If you stay away from food for a while, the next meal you take will usually taste exceptionally delicious.

When your senses are withdrawn for a time, you are able to tune in to the subtler tastes and smells. Yoga suggests that the same is true for all your experiences in the world. If you take the time to withdraw from the world for a little while, you will find that your experiences are more vibrant.

In practice, Pratyahara means paying attention to the sensory impulses you encounter throughout the day, limiting to the extent possible those that are toxic and maximizing those that are nourishing to your body, mind, and soul.

Choose sounds, sensations, sights, tastes, and smells that inspire you. Be aware of and do your best to reduce situations, circumstances, and people who deplete you of your vitality and enthusiasm for life. When it comes to your yoga practice, Pratyahara means defining a space where you are less likely to be distracted by distressing sensations in your environment such as loud music, blaring television shows, and aggravating arguments, so you can bring your awareness to quieter realms within your consciousness. It means taking time on a daily basis to close your eyes so you can settle into more expanded states of awareness through meditation.

The Sixth Branch of Yoga— Dharana

Dharana is the mastery of attention and intention. The world at its essential core is a quantum soup of energy and information. What you actually perceive is a selective act of your attention and interpretation. The difference between an apple and an orange or a rose and a carnation boils down to differences in the quantity and quality of the energy and information that comprise the object of your perception. Through your attention and intention, you freeze the energy and information contained in a fragrant, soft-petaled, thorny-stemmed flower and create a multisensory representation in your awareness that you identify as a rose. Without the unique biology of your human nervous system, the concept of a rose would only exist as a potential.

Whatever you place your attention on grows in importance to you. Whether your attention is on building a business, becoming physically fit, improving a relationship, or developing a spiritual practice, the object of your on is enlivened by your awareness and becomes a more predominant force in your life. By learning to value your attention as a precious commodity, you will be able to consciously create well-being and success in your life. An essential component of yoga is refining your attention in order to facilitate healing and transformation in your body/mind.

Once you activate something with your attention, your intentions have a powerful influence on what things manifest in your life. According to yoga, your intentions have infinite organizing power. Your intention may be to heal an illness, create more love in your life, or become more aware of your own divinity. Simply by becoming clear about your intentions, you will begin to see them actualize in your life. When your awareness is established in being and you have a clear intention, nature rallies to help you fulfill your deepest desires.

Be aware of your intentions. Make a list of the most important things you would like to see unfold in your life. Review them twice daily before you go into meditation. As your mind quiets down, release your intentions, surrendering your desires to the universe. Then pay attention to the clues that arise in your life that are directing you to the fulfillment of your desires. We'll explore attention and intention in greater depth in the next chapter.

The Seventh Branch of Yoga— Dhyana

Dhyana is the development of witnessing awareness. It is the expression of knowing that you are in this world but not of this world. Throughout your life you have experi-

ences, which change moment to moment. Your environment changes, your friends change, your employment
changes, your body changes, your feelings change, your
thoughts change. The only constant in life is perpetual
change. Dhyana is the cultivation of your awareness so
that in the midst of this unending change, you do not lose
your self in the objects of your experience. Although situations, circumstances, people, and things are ever
changing in your life, the aspect of you that is witnessing
these changes is the essence of your being—your soul.

The most direct way to cultivate this state of ever-
present witnessing awareness is through meditation,
during which you learn to observe the thoughts, feelings,
sensations, and sounds that arise in your awareness
without needing to react to them. As you develop this
skill in meditation, you are able to apply it in your
daily life. You learn to stay centered and awake to all
possibilities whenever a challenge arises, so that you are
able to choose the best course of action that will maximize
the chances that your intentions and desires will be fulfilled.

The Eighth Branch of Yoga— Samadhi

Samadhi is the state of being settled in pure, unbounded
awareness. Going beyond time and space, beyond past
and future, beyond individuality, Samadhi is tasting the
realm of eternity and infinity. This is your essential
nature. Immersing yourself in Samadhi on a regular basis
catalyzes the transformation of your internal reference
point from ego to spirit. You perform your actions in the

world as an individual while your inner state is one of a universal being.

This is a state of being in which fear and anxiety do not arise. You surrender your need to take yourself too seriously because you recognize that life is a cosmic play, and like a great actor, you perform your role impeccably but do not lose your real self in the character you're playing. This is the goal of yoga—to know yourself as a spiritual being disguised as a human being, to be established in union and perform action in harmony with the evolutionary flow of life.

We've now explored the map of yoga as elaborated by Patanjali, the great voyager of inner space. In the next chapter, we'll delve into the principles that support the foundation of yoga—the Seven Spiritual Laws that govern the relationship between the body, mind, and soul.

4

The Seven Spiritual Laws of Yoga

If you can cease all restless activity, your integral nature will appear.

—*Lao Tzu*

We have reviewed the theoretical frameworks presented by two of the greatest yogis the world has known, Shankara and Patanjali. These closely related classic approaches remain as the cornerstones of yoga philosophy. In this chapter, we will apply the Seven Spiritual Laws of Success to the principles and practice of yoga. The Seven Spiritual Laws of Success are the laws of nature applied to the human experience. They are the principles through which the unmanifest becomes the manifest; through which spirit becomes the material universe. We believe there is value in applying the seven laws to the practice of yoga because the principles that underlie yoga are the principles that support a life of balance, flexibility, and vitality. The practice of yoga is practice for life. Success in yoga provides a template for success in life.

The seven laws are presented below in a condensed form with a focus on their application to a yogic practice. Each law is associated with a specific mantra whose vibration resonates with the core principle. We encourage you to review the law of the day each morning when you awaken and each evening before bed for a few minutes. Throughout the day, bring the corresponding mantra into your awareness so that the energy of the law resonates within you.

For years, people around the world have begun their days with a review of one of the laws and the intention to implement it throughout the day. We suggest that you focus on the first spiritual law of success on the Sunday of every week. Each subsequent day, put your attention on the next law, ending with the seventh law on Saturday. In this way, you will begin resonating with the millions of other people who are putting their attention on the Seven Spiritual Laws of Success. Let's review each of them as they apply to the practice of yoga.

Day of the Week	Spiritual Law
Sunday	Law of Pure Potentiality
Monday	Law of Giving and Receiving
Tuesday	Law of Karma (or Cause and Effect)
Wednesday	Law of Least Effort
Thursday	Law of Intention and Desire

| Friday | Law of Detachment |
| Saturday | Law of Dharma (or Purpose in Life) |

Law 1. The Law of Pure Potentiality

The first spiritual law of success is the Law of Pure Potentiality, which states that at the core of your being you are pure awareness. This realm of pure awareness is the domain of all possibilities and underlies creativity in all its forms. Pure consciousness is your spiritual essence and the source of your joy in life. The realm of pure potentiality is the home of knowledge, intuition, balance, harmony, and bliss. Giving rise to thoughts, feelings, and actions, it remains undisturbed. This domain is the womb of silence that gives birth to all forms and phenomena in life. It is your essential nature. At your core you are pure potentiality.

The silent ever-present witness is your true Self. The experience of the Self, or *self-referral*, means that your internal reference point is your soul rather than the objects of your experience. The opposite of self-referral is *object-referral*. In object-referral, you are influenced by what is happening outside the Self, which includes situations, circumstances, people, and things. In object-referral, you need and therefore are constantly seeking the approval of others in order to feel comfortable and worthy. Because in object-referral your thoughts and behavior are always in anticipation of a response, it is a fear-based state of being.

The ego is your internal reference in the state of object-referral. The ego, however, is not who you really are. Rather, it is your social mask, the roles you are playing. At one moment you play the role of friend, in the next the antagonist. You play the role of child in the presence of your parents and the role of parent when you are with your children. You play one role when speaking with your supervisor and another with those you supervise.

Your social mask thrives on approval, strives to control, and is sustained by power. The corollary of this is that your ego lives in fear of losing approval, control, and power.

But your true Self, your soul, is completely free of these things. It is immune to criticism, fears no challenge, and feels neither beneath nor above anyone. Your soul recognizes at its deepest level that everyone else is the same Self in different disguises.

During the practice of yoga, the Law of Pure Potentiality reminds us that every movement emerges from the silent field of infinite possibility. The more powerful the silence, the more effective the movement. Every movement is a vibration, a wave on the ocean of life. The deeper the connection to the depths of the ocean, the more powerful is the wave that arises.

While practicing your yoga poses, bring your attention back to the silent space within you between every movement and every posture. Remain in a state of mindful witnessing as you perform each pose, cultivating the experience of having your awareness in this nonlocalized domain of pure potentiality as you engage in activities localized in time and space.

Enliven the Law of Pure Potentiality while performing yoga poses and throughout your day by taking the time to do the following three things:

1. Cultivate stillness in your body and mind. Between poses and between movements, bring your attention to the quiet stillness within you. After performing your set of yoga postures, sit alone in silent meditation for approximately twenty minutes. By quieting the mind in meditation, you will learn to directly experience the field of pure awareness, where everything is inseparably connected with everything else.

2. During your postures and during each day, practice shifting into a witnessing mode of awareness. Observe from the inner stillness of your soul the dynamic activity of the world. Take time each day to commune with nature and silently witness the intelligence within every living thing. Watch a sunset, listen to the sound of the ocean or a stream, or simply smell the scent of a flower. From the peace of your inner silence and through your communion with nature, you will experience joy and reverence for the eternal movement of life in all its manifestations.

3. Practice nonjudgment. While performing your yoga postures, relinquish the need to judge your ability. Begin each session with the statement, "Today, I shall judge nothing that occurs," and remind yourself that self-acceptance is the source and goal of yoga. When you are constantly making judgments, including of yourself, as things being right or wrong, good or bad, you create turbulence in your internal dialogue, which constricts the flow of energy between you and the field of pure potentiality. Nonjudgment cultivates silence in the mind, which gives you direct access to the field of pure potentiality.

Memorize the mantra, whose vibratory qualities resonate with the Law of Pure Potentiality, and silently repeat it a few times throughout the day to remind you that your essential nature is pure potentiality.

Om Bhavam Namah
I am absolute existence

Law 2.   The Law of Giving and Receiving

The second spiritual law of success is the Law of Giving and Receiving, which states that the universe operates through dynamic exchange. Your body is in constant and dynamic exchange with the body of the universe. Your mind is dynamically interacting with the mind of the cosmos. Life is the flow of all the elements and forces that comprise the field of existence. The harmonious exchange between your physical body and the physical universe and between your personal mind and the collective mind is expressed as the Law of Giving and Receiving. Because your body, your mind, and the universe are in constant and dynamic exchange, stopping the circulation of energy is like stopping the flow of blood. Whenever blood stops flowing, it begins to clot, to coagulate. Whenever a river stops flowing, it begins to stagnate. This is why you must be open to giving and receiving in order to keep the life force circulating within you.

The most important thing is the intention behind your giving and receiving. The intention should always be to create happiness for the giver and the receiver, because happiness is life-supporting and life-sustaining. The return is proportional to the giving when it is unconditional and from the heart. This is why the act of giving has to be joyful—the frame of mind has to be one in which you feel joy in the very act of giving. Then the energy behind the giving increases many times over.

During your yoga practice, the Law of Giving and Receiving is lively in every breath you take. With each inhalation and exhalation, you are exchanging ten billion trillion atoms with your environment. Right now, take as deep a breath as you possibly can and hold it. Hold it as long as you can, and notice how uncomfortable you begin to feel when you are holding onto something that is meant to be released. Now, exhale as fully as you can and hold your breath with your lungs fully emptied. Again, feel the discomfort that arises when you are resisting taking in something that you need. Whenever you resist the Law of Giving and Receiving, your mind becomes anxious and your body becomes uncomfortable.

With every pose you assume, complementary pairs of muscles are contracting and relaxing, holding and releasing in accordance with the Law of Giving and Receiving. When the life force is flowing freely through your body/mind, you are in natural alignment with the generosity and receptivity of the universe.

Make the commitment to put the second law of success into effect in your yoga practice by taking the following three steps:

1. During your yoga poses, maintain breathing awareness, effortlessly exchanging air with your environment through the inflow and outflow of your

breath. Anytime throughout the day that you feel resistance in your body because things are not going the way you think they should, bring your attention to your breath and use it to regain your sense of effortless receiving and releasing.

2.   Cultivate the sense of gratitude for the gifts you have in your life. During your yoga practice, tune into the life force that is circulating through your body and be grateful for the opportunity to experience life through a human mind and body. Enjoy the sensation of your body contracting and expanding as your move through your postures. Celebrate your physical manifestation that enables your soul to express its meaning and purpose in life. Celebrate the very improbability of your existence.

Our beloved teacher Brahmananda Saraswati once said that it might take a million incarnations until you gain a human nervous system; if you do not use it to remember and rejoice in your sacred nature, you have traded a diamond for a head of lettuce.

3.   During your practice of yoga have the intention of surrendering to the needs of your body. Rather than forcing your will upon your body to attain a specific pose, practice listening to the needs of your muscles and joints. The impulse to give flows naturally from the experience of gratitude. You will find that through this subtle shift in your attitude, challenging postures are more easily achieved.

Outside of your asana practice have the intention to give something to everyone you come into contact with during the day. It might be a kind word, a compliment, a smile, a prayer, or a small gift. Similarly, be open to receiving the gifts that come to you during the day. They may be gifts from nature, such as the songs of birds, a spring shower, a rainbow, or a beautiful sunset. They may be gifts from people in your life—a warm embrace, a kind gesture, a helpful suggestion. Make the commitment to enliven the Law of Giving and Receiving by taking every opportunity to circulate love, caring, affection, appreciation, and acceptance.

Learn the mantra whose vibratory qualities resonate with the Law of Giving and Receiving, and repeat it silently to yourself whenever you find yourself restricting the flow of giving and receiving in your life.

Om Vardhanam Namah
I am the nourisher of the universe

Law 3. The Law of Karma (or Cause and Effect)

The third spiritual law of success pertains to *karma*, or cause and effect. Every action we take generates a force of energy that returns to us in kind—as we sow, so we reap. When we consciously choose actions that bring happiness and success to others, the fruit of our karma is happiness and success.

Although many people misinterpret the Law of Karma as imprisoning us in a cycle of unending reactivity, it is actually an assertion of human freedom. Karma implies the action of conscious choice-making for we are all infinite choice makers. In every moment of your existence, the real you resides in the field of pure potentiality where you have access to unlimited choices. Some of these choices are made consciously, while most are made unconsciously. The best way to understand and maximize the use of karmic law is to become consciously aware of the choices you make in every moment.

Whether you like it or not, everything that is happening at this moment is a result of the choices you've made in the past. When you make choices unconsciously, you don't think they are choices, and yet they are. If you step back a moment and witness the choices you are making, then in just this act of witnessing you take the process from the unconscious into the conscious realm. In every situation, there is one choice out of the many available that will create happiness for you as well as for those around you. And when you make that one choice it will nourish you and everyone else influenced by that action.

Applied to your practice of yoga, the Law of Karma is demonstrated as you consciously move through your postures aware of how there is a reaction for every action you execute. If in your impatience you force yourself into a pose that you are not fully ready to perform, your body/ mind will react, and the consequences of your straining will generate feelings of strain within you. On the other hand, when you move gracefully into the limits of each pose with an attitude of gentleness and finesse, your body/mind responds with effortlessness and ease.

Notice that by slowing down your movements, you become more aware of the karmic consequences of your choices. If your body is unusually uncomfortable the morning after a yoga session, it is most likely the result of your ignoring the Law of Karma. You probably pushed too hard, making a less than ideal choice, and the karmic cost is your discomfort.

Karma presents itself in your present by reminding you of your past. Choosing more consciously from the witnessing realm of quiet awareness, you make karma-free choices.

Put the Law of Karma into effect in your yoga practice and your life so that you make the most evolutionary choices. Commit yourself to the following three steps:

1. As you move through your yoga practice, witness the choices you make in each moment. In the witnessing of your choices, you will bring them into your conscious awareness. Be fully present in this moment and your next moment will not carry the consequences of the prior one. The best way to prepare for any moment in the future is to be fully conscious in the present.

2. As you make your choice about how to move through resistance in your poses, ask yourself two questions: "What are the consequences of the choice I'm making?" and "Will this choice bring comfort?" When you make your choices outside of your practice of yoga, ask yourself, "Which choice is most likely to bring happiness and fulfillment to me and to those affected by my choice?"

3. Then listen to your heart for guidance and be guided by its message of comfort or discomfort. Your heart is the junction point between your mind and your body. If the choice feels comfortable in your body, move into it with confidence. If the choice

feels uncomfortable, pause and see the consequences of your action with your inner vision. Honoring the guidance that is provided by your body's intelligence will help you make the most evolutionary choices for yourself and those in your life.

Become familiar with the mantra whose vibratory qualities resonate with the Law of Karma and repeat it to yourself when you are making karmically significant choices. Thinking the mantra will remind you to listen to your body so your choice will be most likely to provide you with greater comfort and joy.

Om Kriyam Namah
My actions are aligned with cosmic law

Law 4. The Law of Least Effort

The Law of Least Effort states that nature's intelligence functions with effortless ease. If you look at the ebb and flow of the tides, the blossoming of a flower, or the movement of the stars, you do not see nature straining. There is rhythm and balance in the natural world, and when you are in harmony with nature, you can make use of the Law of Least Effort by minimizing your effort and maximizing your effect.

When a Newtonian model of the world predominated in our collective awareness, the principles of force and effort were dominant. But in our modern era, when quantum physics provides the most comprehensive model of how the universe works, there is no place for force and effort. Rather, timing and finesse are the tools for transformation in a world that is understood as the expression of an underlying field of energy and information. Stated simply, the Law of Least Effort tells us that we can do less and accomplish more.

Nature is held together by the energy of love, and least effort is expended when your actions are motivated by love. When your soul is your internal reference point, you can harness the power of love and use the energy creatively for healing, transformation, and evolution.

The Law of Least Effort is of immeasurable value during the practice of yoga. Yoga is the antidote to the prescription "no pain, no gain." The greatest benefits of yoga come from relaxing into a pose, rather than forcing your body into it. When moving into a flexibility pose, find the point of resistance. Rather than muscling your way through this point, breathe into the resistance—surrender into the resistance—and you will find yourself extending your reach and enhancing your flexibility. Stay present with your full awareness in your body and engage an attitude of surrender. In yoga as in life, patience is a virtue. In yoga, the more you are able to embrace rather than fight your limitations and vulnerabilities, the less limits they hold and the more balance and energy you experience.

To enliven the Law of Least Effort in your yoga practice and in your life, make a commitment to the following three steps:

1. Practice acceptance. During your yoga practice, accept your body the way it is. Although you may have intention for it to change in some way, accept that how it is now is exactly as it should be, because

the universe is as it should be. Give up your need to struggle against the whole universe by struggling against this moment. By acknowledging each situation as it exists, you are in the best position to help evolve it to a new level.

In your daily life, practice accepting people as they are and circumstances as they occur, understanding that every moment in your life is the consequence of every prior choice you've made. Rather than resisting who or what is currently in your life, practice acceptance of what is present and reinforce your commitment to make more conscious choices from this moment on.

2. Having accepted things as they are, take responsibility for the challenge you are facing. As applied to your yoga practice, this means making the commitment to nurture your body through appropriate exercise and nutrition. If you are seeking to change your body in a positive way, taking responsibility does not mean indulging in blame for the state of your body now. Remember that every challenge is an opportunity in disguise, and this alertness to opportunity allows you to take this moment and transform it for greater benefit.

3. Establish your awareness in defenselessness. Do not waste your life energy defending your point of view or attempting to convince others. Remain open to all points of view without rigidly attaching yourself to any one of them.

The third principle is of particular relevance to your yoga practice. There are many different schools of yoga without one right way. Every teacher and every system has its own variations on postures, pace, style, and intensity. As a system dedicated to awakening flexibility in body, mind, and spirit, yoga can accommodate and celebrate the many diverse approaches that have developed over past centuries.

Experiment for yourself with different approaches and find the style that fits best with your needs at a given time of your life. The right yoga system for you is the one that enhances your vitality and flexibility. Commit yourself to the Law of Least Effort and you will cease wasting your vital energy in friction and conflict. Liberated, this energy becomes available to you for creativity, personal growth, and healing.

Whenever you find yourself forcing an outcome that is not ready to manifest, remember the Law of Least Effort. Introduce the mantra that resonates with the principle that you can accomplish more by doing less if you are not wasting energy by struggling and straining.

Om Daksham Namah
My actions achieve maximal benefit
with minimal effort

Law 5.   The Law of Intention and Desire

The fifth spiritual law of success is the Law of Intention and Desire, which is based upon the recognition that at the level of the quantum field there is nothing other than energy and information. This quantum field, which is really just another name for the field of pure potentiality, is influenced by intention and desire.

As a human being, you experience the quantum field subjectively as your own thoughts, feelings, memories, desires, needs, expectations, fantasies, and beliefs. You experience the same field objectively as your physical body and the physical world. At the level of the field, the collection of thoughts called your mind and the collection of molecules called your body are different disguises of the same underlying reality. The ancient yogic sages had an expression for this realization, "*Tat Tvam Asi*," which translates as, "I am that, you are that, all this is that, and that's all there is."

If you accept that your personal body is not separate from the body of the universe, then by consciously changing the energy and informational content of your own body, you can influence the energy and information of your extended body—your environment, your world. This influence is activated by two qualities inherent in consciousness: *attention* and *intention*. Attention enlivens while intention transforms.

If you want something to grow stronger in your life, direct more of your attention to it. If you want something to diminish in your life, withdraw your attention from it. Intention, on the other hand, catalyzes the transformation of energy and information into new forms and expressions. According to ancient yogic principles, your intention has organizing power.

Accomplished yogis are masters of attention and intention. They can influence components of their physiology in ways that modern science used to think were impossible. Yogis can raise and lower their blood pressure, speed up or slow down their heart rates, increase or decrease their body temperature, and bring their respiratory system and metabolic activity to almost imperceptible levels. In chapter 5, we will show you how to use your attention and intention for healing and transformation. As you become increasingly adept at governing your own body through the Law of Intention and Desire, you will also experience your intentions being increasingly supported by nature.

You can learn to harness the power of the Law of Intention and Desire in your yoga practice and in your life by following these three steps:

1.   Be clear about your intentions and desires. On a regular basis, take the time to write down a list of those things you would like to see manifest in your life. Review your intentions and desires prior to beginning your yoga practice and prior to your time of silent meditation. Modify your list as your desires are fulfilled or transformed and observe how your intentions and desires evolve. When you take the time to document what you desire in your heart and mind, you accelerate the process of manifesting your desires in the world.

2.   Even as you bring your intentions and desires into conscious awareness, surrender the outcome to nature. Cultivate an attitude of trusting that when things are not going exactly the way you intend them to, there is a grander design at work. You can probably identify times in your life when things were not going according to your plan, only to realize later that something better was waiting for you around the corner.

When performing your yoga poses, maintain this inner attitude of surrender. Attend to and release your intentions as you move through your postures and watch the result in your yoga practice and in your life.

3. Remind yourself to practice present moment awareness in all your actions. Do not allow any obstacles to consume or dissipate the quality of your attention in the present moment. As you engage in a pose, be fully in the present, remembering that being in the moment empowers your most cherished intentions and desires.

As you energize your intentions and desires with your attention, introduce the mantra that resonates with the Law of Intention and Desire.

Om Ritam Namah
My intentions and desires are supported
by cosmic intelligence

Law 6.   The Law of Detachment

The sixth spiritual law of success is the Law of Detachment, which reveals a great paradox of life. In order to acquire something in this world, you have to relinquish your attachment to it. This doesn't mean you give up the intention to fulfill your desire—you simply give up your attachment to the outcome.

Attachment is based on fear and insecurity. When you forget that the only genuine source of security is your true self, you begin believing that you need something outside yourself in order to be happy. You may believe that a certain amount of money in the bank, paying off the mortgage on your house, obtaining a luxury car, losing ten pounds, or purchasing a new outfit may result in greater feelings of security within yourself. Unfortunately, whenever your happiness is based upon something other than your true Self, insecurity arises because you know at a deep level of your being that whatever is bringing you happiness can be lost and therefore has the potential to bring you pain.

According to the principles of yoga, the only true security comes from your willingness to embrace the unknown, the realm of uncertainty. By relinquishing your attachment to the known, you step into the field of pure potentiality in which the wisdom of uncertainty is factored into all your choices. Practicing detachment and embracing uncertainty, you relinquish your need to hold on to the past, which is the only thing that is known. Being open to what is happening rather than trying to control how things unfold, you experience the excitement, adventure, exhilaration, and mystery of life.

Applied to your practice of yoga, the Law of Detachment encourages you to relinquish your attachment to an idealized pose. Rather than seeking only to achieve the perfect posture, have the intention for your practice to awaken deeper and more expanded levels of awareness within you. By relinquishing your attachment to an idealized form and allowing your awareness to embrace the essence of yoga, your body will naturally release its resistance, increase its flexibility, and will improve as a side benefit for your detachment.

Yoga is not a competitive sport, and you will not achieve integration of body, mind, and spirit through force and effort. Rather, yoga is a system of mindful surrender.

The practice of yoga accomplishes its goal of union through attention and intention—through the conscious release of conflict and struggle. This is the essence of the Law of Detachment. Have your intentions clearly in your awareness while you maintain an attitude of *Thy will be done*. The coexistence of these apparently contradictory forces—intention and detachment—cultivates the flexibility that enables you to fulfill all your goals in life.

Put the Law of Detachment into effect in your yoga practice and in your life by making a commitment to the following three steps:

1. Practice detachment. The goal of yoga is flexibility, for which detachment is an essential feature. Detachment and flexibility go hand in hand. Attachment breeds rigidity. Commit not to rigidly impose your ideas of how things should be. Allow yourself and those around you the freedom to be natural. Notice that when you force solutions on problems, you often create new problems that did not previously exist. Remind yourself to engage in everything with detached involvement.

2. Embrace uncertainty as an essential ingredient of your experience and watch how creative solutions to problems spontaneously emerge out of chaos. Cultivate an attitude of curiosity and innocence as you live your life and notice how a deep inner security develops within you, independent of things around you.

3. Surrender to the field of pure potentiality. Combine your focused intention with detachment from

the outcome and observe how easily you are able to fulfill your desires while maintaining your center, even in the midst of confusion and turbulence.

Introduce the mantra that resonates with the Law of Detachment to remind you to relinquish your need to control, thereby allowing creative solutions to emerge from the wisdom of uncertainty.

Om Anandham Namah
My actions are blissfully free from
attachment to outcome

Law 7. The Law of Dharma (or Purpose in Life)

The seventh spiritual law is the Law of Dharma, which states that every sentient being has a purpose in life. You have unique abilities and your own way of expressing them. There are needs in this world for which your specific talents are ideally suited, and when the world's needs are matched with the creative expression of your talents, your purpose—your dharma—is realized.

To be in dharma, your life force must flow effortlessly without interference. The practice of yoga provides a direct mechanism to release energy blockages in your body. When obstacles to the flow of your vital energy are removed, you become capable of expressing more expanded aspects of your self. Increasing compassion, wisdom, and playfulness are evidence that your life is flowing in accordance with the Law of Dharma.

There are three major components to the Law of

Dharma. The first is that your ultimate purpose is to discover your higher Self. Pursue the god or goddess inside you that wants to express the sacred purpose for which you were born. Awaken to the unbounded, eternal witnessing awareness that is the essence of who you are and know yourself as a timeless, eternal Being in the midst of time-bound experience.

The second component of the Law of Dharma is to acknowledge and express your unique talents. Take the time to honor your innate gifts by making a list of those things that you do well. One way to connect with your dharma is to consider those things that you really love to do. Make a list of the things that bring joy to you and to others while you are doing them. It might be singing, playing the piano, teaching gymnastics, or cooking. You may be naturally good at deep listening or caring for those in need. Whatever your unique talents may be, expressing them brings happiness and satisfaction to you and to others. When you are in the flow of your dharma, expressing your unique talents, time loses its hold on you and you enter into timeless awareness.

The third component of dharma is serving others. True dharmic actions naturally bring benefit both to you and to those affected by your actions.

The inner dialogue of a person in his or her dharma is, "How can I serve?" and "How can I help?" The answers to these questions will allow you to serve your fellow human beings with love and compassion. Expressing your gifts in service to others is the highest expression of the Law of Dharma. When your creative expressions match the needs of your fellow humans, abundance flows into your life.

Yoga is action in accordance with dharma. Moving

your body with awareness and impeccability is the essence of a life in harmony with the laws of nature. Every cell, tissue, and organ in your body has its dharma, which is to perform its unique function while supporting the wholeness of the body. The digestive tract performs its job of secreting gastric juices, moving food along its pathway, absorbing nutrients, and eliminating toxins. The endocrine system secretes its vital hormones that regulate metabolism, reproduction, growth, and repair. The circulatory system regulates blood pressure and cardiac output. While each of these systems has its specific role to perform, the essential purpose of their existence is to support the whole physiology.

Your practice of yoga supports the dharma of your body. When life energy is flowing effortlessly through every cell, tissue, and organ, the dharma of each is being fulfilled. When as a result of the flexibility, balance, and strength gained during your yoga practice you are effortlessly able to express your talents in the world, you are aligned with the Law of Dharma. When you allow the intelligence and vital energy of nature to flow through you, you are reminded of your highest purpose—serving the world and supporting the evolutionary flow of life.

Put the Law of Dharma into effect in your yoga practice and in your life by commiting to the following three steps:

1. Pay attention to the quiet stillness within you that animates your body and mind. During your yoga practice and during the day, bring your attention to the silent witness that observes your thoughts and actions.

2. Become aware of your unique talents and those things you love to do while expressing your unique talents. In your practice of yoga, notice the postures that you enter into easily and use this information to become more intimate with your nature. Some people are naturally flexible, some have inherently good muscle strength, while others have innately good balance. Celebrate your natural talents even as you strive to develop other ones in yoga and in your life.

3. Cultivate an inner conversation of helping and serving. When your intentions behind every action are to align with dharma, your actions will be effortless and successful. By asking the questions, How can I help? and How can I serve? you will fulfill your deeper purpose in life.

Use the mantra that resonates with the Law of Dharma is to remind you of the Law of Dharma, particularly when you are experiencing struggle and strife. Using the mantra will help shift your inner conversation from What's in it for me? to How can I help?

Om Varunam Namah
My life is in harmony with cosmic law

Implement Your Insights

So far we have explored the theory and philosophy of yoga. Yoga is as much a science of action as it is a way of thinking about life. In the next chapters, we will present the essential technologies that when practiced spontaneously implement the theory of yoga into the experience of life. Meditation, regulating the life force, learning to hold and circulate energy, and moving with awareness are the fundamental technologies that need to be mastered for you to gain the full benefits of yoga on the level of your body, your mind, and your soul.

PART II

Meditation and Breathing

5

Meditation
Calming a Turbulent Mind

Empty the cup.

—*Zen master Nan-in*

Your mind is a thought-generating organ. Thought forms perpetually arise in your awareness. If you try to stop your thoughts with the intention of creating stillness in your mind, your mental activity may quiet for a few moments, but it will almost certainly start up again at full speed.

The activity in your mind is communicated to every cell in your body. When your mind is turbulent, your messenger molecules communicate turbulence to your cells, tissues, and organs. If you can quiet your mind, you can send messages of peace and harmony to every cell in your body. To experience the real essence of yoga—the full integration of body, mind, and spirit—you need to develop the ability to calm your mental turbulence.

A thought is a packet of energy and information. According to yoga, all thoughts can be classified as either memories or desires. When your mind is active, you are either thinking about something that happened in the past or are anticipating something occurring in the future. The Sanskrit word for *memory* or *past impression* is *sanskara*, while the word for *desire* is *vasana*.

Impressions give rise to desires. If you see an advertisement for a flashy car, a tropical vacation spot, or a designer dress, an impression is laid down in your mind that may give rise to a desire. As a result of this desire, you are compelled to take some new action, such as going to a car dealership, calling your travel agent, or visiting your local boutique.

The action that emerges from the desire is called *karma*. This endless cycle of impressions giving rise to desires giving rise to actions resulting in new impressions is the circuitry that keeps your mind perpetually active. We can think of this circuit of sanskara, vasana, and karma as the software of your soul. As long as you are thinking, your mind is churning through the cycle of action . . . impression . . . desire . . . action . . . impression . . . desire . . . action.

Meditation is the technology that enables you temporarily to escape from this cycle. Through the process of gently focusing your attention (known in yoga as *Dharana*) while innocently witnessing the thought forms that come and go in your mind (*Dhyana*), you enter into the gap between thoughts, glimpsing the domain of unbounded awareness (*Samadhi*). Taking your mind from constricted to expanded awareness, meditation offers the most direct path to awakening the Law of Pure Potentiality in your life.

Your choices are limited while your mind is engaged in a particular memory or desire. People frequently get caught in habitual ruts of thinking, believing that they are stuck in a situation because they cannot imagine any other possibilities. Accessing the field of pure potentiality by going beyond conditioning through meditation opens up creative possibilities that previously were unavailable.

Meditation can take many different forms, but there is a common theme. In every technique of meditation, the process takes you out of the conditioned mind and opens up access to the nonconditioned mind. This is accomplished by experiencing a thought in its less distinct, more refined aspects until eventually you experience the thought as it emerges from the nonlocal field of your awareness. As you become increasingly familiar with the experience of thoughts condensing from consciousness, your identity begins shifting from your mind to your soul.

You can focus on and refine your perception of objects in any sensory modality. You can use music, chanting, drumming, or the sound of your own breath as a focus of your attention in meditation. You can use visual symbols, a candle flame, pictures of people you love, or a sunset to expand your consciousness. You can go from local to nonlocal awareness through the sense of touch—from therapeutic massage to sexual rapture. You can even momentarily go beyond time and space through the sense of taste and smell.

For every experience in the mind, it is possible to refine that experience so your awareness is less constricted and more expanded. This expanded state of mind is the ultimate expression of the Law of Pure Potentiality, for all possibilities reside in and emerge from this field of unbounded awareness.

Before it arises in your mind, a thought is in this domain of consciousness that is transcendent to thought, a domain accessible through meditation. An ancient powerful meditation technique involves asking the question, Who is having these thoughts? By repeated inquiry, you reach the awareness that thoughts arise from a deeper domain of awareness over which your mind really has no control.

In the yoga tradition, meditation classically involves the use of a mantra or primordial sound. The word *mantra* means "instrument or vehicle of the mind." Mantras are used to take your awareness from engagement in the changing realm of life to immersion in the expanded state of being that is beyond beginnings and endings. These vibrations, used for thousands of years to quiet mental activity, are pleasing, resonant sounds that do not have specific meanings to keep your mind active. The mind stays active through the process of association. If you listen to your mind, it may sound like this:

> *I need to reduce my credit card debt . . . I really didn't need to buy that sweater last week . . . I did need something to wear to Stan's party . . . The food was really great . . . I wish I hadn't eaten so much . . . I am definitely going to start exercising next week . . . I am going to try to get Tanya to go out with me . . . I wonder if she got the job she was applying for . . . and on . . . and on . . . and on . . .*

Introducing a mantra temporarily interrupts the incessant association process that keeps the mind active. Introducing a thought that does not carry meaning momentarily breaks the cycle and allows you to glimpse the silent space between your thoughts. This starts the transformation of your identity from mind to spirit.

The best-known mantra is the sound *Aum* or *Om*, traditionally said to be the sound the universe makes when it manifests from potential to perceptual. Using the sound that represents the junction point between local and nonlocal can take your awareness back to the field of awareness that gives rise to the mind.

At the Chopra Center, we teach a mantra meditation technique called Primordial Sound Meditation, which assigns a person one of 108 mantras based upon the date and place of a person's birth. This requires personalized instruction, which is available through our certified meditation instructors in most cities throughout the world.

According to the theory that underlies Primordial Sound Meditation, the universe expresses a different vibratory frequency at different times during the day. You can appreciate this principle by considering how the environment feels different at dawn from the way it does at high noon or at dusk. Over the course of a lunar month, the "sound" of the world changes about 108 times. One of these 108 sounds is assigned based upon the time, date, and place of a person's birth. This primordial sound or mantra is said to represent the sound of the cosmos at the doorway between potentiality and individuality because until we emerge through the birth canal we are potential human beings. This primordial sound can be used as a meditation vehicle to take you back through the doorway from individuality to universality—the ultimate goal of meditation.

Chakra Meditation

A different type of meditation involves intoning mantras aloud to create a healing resonance in the mind and body. There are mantras associated with each of the seven energy centers in the body, known as chakras. The chakras are major junction points between consciousness and the body, and each one is associated with a specific vibration. Envisioned by the ancient seers as wheels or vortices of life force, they sometimes have been associated with major neural networks or hormonal systems.

Chakra	Neural Association	Hormonal Association
First—Root	Sacral plexus	Adrenal glands
Second— Creativity	Lumbar plexus	Reproductive glands
Third—Energy	Solar plexus	Pancreas (insulin)
Fourth—Heart	Cardiac plexus	Thymus gland
Fifth— Expression	Cervical plexus	Thyroid gland
Sixth—Intuition	Carotid plexus	Pituitary gland
Seventh— Consciousness	Cerebral cortex	Pineal gland

Each center identifies a core human need. When the center is open, the energy that flows through the chakra allows you to meet those needs more effortlessly. If there is a blockage in one area of the body/mind system, energy becomes stagnant and your intentions are more difficult to actualize. You can activate each center by putting your attention in the location of the chakra and sounding the associated mantra aloud.

To begin this meditation, sit comfortably with your spine upright. Close your eyes and visualize the site of the energy center you wish to focus on. Take a deep breath, and on the inhalation, chant the mantra in one long syllable. Feel the sensations in your body and notice the sense of alert calm in your mind after each mantra. Envision energy flowing effortlessly from the base of your spine through the different energy centers and rising up through the top of your head. Notice how you feel in the meditation and how it affects you when you return to your active life.

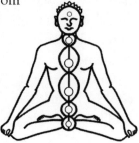

The First Center: Root Chakra

The root chakra, known in Sanskrit as *Muladhara*, is located at the base of the spine. It governs your most basic survival needs. When energy is flowing freely through this center, you have confidence that you can meet your core needs without struggle. When there is blockage in this area, you will tend to experience anxiety and worry.

The Law of Karma governs the first energy center. On the physical plane, every action you perform results in a corresponding reaction. To maximize the possibility that your actions generate evolutionary reactions, you can use your body as a choice-determining instrument. Consider the possibilities in front of you and listen to the signals from your body. These sensations generating from the root chakra are either comfortable or uncomfortable.

Your body evaluates every possible decision in terms of its likelihood to meet your needs for safety or increase the level of threat you experience. The first chakra, which connects you with the earth, provides essential information as to the potential nourishment or toxicity that is available to you as a result of the actions you are taking. Keeping energy open and flowing in this source chakra is key to both physical and emotional abundance.

The color for this energy center is red. It is associated with the element earth and the sense of smell.

The mantra for the first chakra is *Lam*.

The Second Center: Creativity Chakra

The second chakra, called *Svadhisthana*, is associated with creativity in all its expressions. It is located in the area of your sexual organs, and the energy of this center can be used for biological reproduction. When channeled into higher energy centers, it fuels the creative force that enables you to paint a beautiful picture, write a novel, play music, build a business, or create a life of love and abundance.

The Law of Least Effort is lively in the second chakra.

When your vital energy is flowing through your center or creativity, you cocreate your life.

The solution to every problem is rarely on the level of the problem. Rather, it comes from a deeper domain of creativity. Creativity is the process of taking the same raw material and creating different contexts and relationships between the components. When a painter creates a masterpiece of art, she weaves the pigments in a way that results in a unique creation. When a composer creates a new piece of music, he is using the same notes in a new relationship with each other, resulting in the emergence of something that did not exist before. A novelist creates a new relationship between letters and words, enabling a story to manifest that had not previously existed.

When you are aligned with your creative juices, the expressions that emerge arise effortlessly. The second chakra utilizes the raw material of the root chakra to create the world anew each day.

The color for the second energy center is orange. It is associated with the element of water and the sense of taste.

The mantra for the second chakra is *Vam.*

The Third Center: Energy Chakra

The third chakra, *Manipura*, is localized in your solar plexus. It is the seat of your power in the world. When this center is open and flowing, you are capable of translating your intentions and desires into manifestation. When it is blocked, you feel frustrated and ineffectual.

The seeds of intentions and desires reside in your personal soul. Nourishing the seeds you wish to germinate with your attention will lead to their full expression. The Law of Intention and Desire governs the third chakra. It is important to be clear about your intentions so you are not surprised when they bear fruit. The process of manifesting your desires is first to bring them into consciousness, then expand your awareness through meditation, then release your intentions and detach from the outcome.

You can control your actions, but you cannot control the fruit of your actions. Keep your life energy flowing freely through your third chakra and the light and heat of your intentions will radiate to the world.

The color for the third energy center is yellow like the sun. It is associated with the element of fire and the sense of sight.

The mantra to clear and enliven the third chakra is *Ram.*

The Fourth Center: Heart Chakra

The fourth chakra represents the unifying energy of love and compassion. Known as *Anahata*, the heart chakra is dedicated to overcoming separation and division. When the heart center is blocked, there is a sense of alienation from others. When the heart center is open and flowing, you feel connected at a deep level to all beings in your life.

The Law of Giving and Receiving governs the heart chakra. Love can take many different forms at different stages of life. The love of a child for his mother is different from a mother's love for her child. A friend's love is different from a passionate lover's love or the love of a student for his teacher. The common thread in each of these expressions of love is the impulse to unify—

to overcome separation. This is the nature of the heart.

The Law of Giving and Receiving as expressed through the fourth chakra establishes the principle that the heart is the organ that circulates love. The relationship between the physical heart and the emotional heart is more than metaphorical. Studies have shown that in patients with recent heart attacks, men who believe that their spouses love them suffer fewer complications and have better outcomes then men who are in conflicted marriages. People who perceive the world as hostile have a higher risk of premature heart attacks than those who feel the world is a nurturing place. Just the simple act of a cardiac nurse calling to check on the well-being of patients recently discharged from a coronary care unit can reduce the risk of rehospitalization.

Every act of giving is simultaneously an act of receiving. Each time you welcome a gift into your life you are providing the opportunity for someone to give. Just as a healthy physical heart receives blood from the periphery which it then oxygenates and pumps back out, your emotional heart stays healthy by receiving and giving love in all its forms.

The color of the fourth energy center is green. When flowing, it is the green of nourishment; when congested, it can be green with envy. It is associated with the element of air and the sense of touch.

The mantra that awakens the fourth chakra is *Yum*.

The Fifth Center: Expression Chakra

The throat chakra, called *Vishuddha* in Sanskrit, is the center of expression. When it is open and flowing, you have the confidence that you are capable of communicating your needs. When the fifth chakra is obstructed, a person will often feel that he is not being heard. To feel alive and empowered, it is important that this energy center is clear. Energy blockages in this area are often associated with thyroid problems or chronic neck pain.

The Law of Detachment governs the throat chakra. An open fifth chakra enables you to express your truth without concern for censors or critics. This does not mean you say things that are intentionally hurtful or insensitive. On the contrary, people with open centers of communication are skillful in expressing their needs in ways that are life-supporting. Anxiety over how people will react to your views does not arise when energy is flowing freely through the chakra of expression.

The Law of Detachment reminds you that you can choose your words and actions, but you cannot control the response to your words and actions. When your intentions are clear and your heart is open, you will spontaneously demonstrate right speech, trusting that the universe will handle the details.

The color of the fifth energy center is blue. It is associated with the elements of ether or space and the sense of hearing.

The mantra to open the fifth chakra is *Hum*.

The Sixth Center: Intuition Chakra

The sixth energy center is sometimes known as the third eye. Located in the forehead, *Ajna*, as it is known in Sanskrit, is the center of insight and intuition. When this center is open, you have a deep sense of connection to your inner voice and feel guided in your choices. When it is blocked, there is a sense of self-doubt and distrust. The opening of this chakra is usually associated with a clear sense of connection to one's dharma or purpose in life.

The Law of Dharma or Purpose in Life governs the sixth chakra. You have within you a wise voice guiding you to express the highest aspects of your nature. Listen to this inner still voice, which is guiding you to manifest your full potential. Quiet the internal turbulence that is filled with the voices of others so you can identify the sound of your own soul. It has only one desire—for you to remember your essential nature as a spark of the divine.

The color of the sixth energy center is indigo. It is associated with extrasensory perceptual abilities such as clairvoyance, clairaudience, and remote viewing. The sense is inner sound, independent of outside vibrations.

The mantra to awaken the sixth chakra is *Sham*.

The Seventh Center: Consciousness Chakra

This center, known as *Sahaswara*, is visualized as a lotus flower at the crown of the head. When the lotus unfolds its petals, the memory of wholeness is restored. You remember that your essential nature is unbounded and that you are spirit in disguise as a person. This is the full expression of yoga—the unification of being with action, of universality with individuality.

The Law of Pure Potentiality governs the seventh chakra. When your roots are receiving nourishment from the earth in the first chakra, your creative juices are flowing in the second, your intentions are empowered in the third, your heart is open and exchanging love with those around you in the fourth, you are spontaneously expressing your highest self in the fifth, and you are in touch with your inner voice in the sixth, then energy moves into the crown chakra and you remember your essential nature as infinite and unbounded. The thousand-petaled lotus flower unfolds and you know yourself as a spiritual being temporarily localized to a body and mind.

As you recognize the universality underlying your individuality, you gain access to your full potential. Your identity shifts from local to nonlocal, from constricted to expanded. Fear and anxiety dissipate because you lose your attachment to specific outcomes, trusting that the universe is unfolding in the most evolutionary way possible.

The color of the seventh energy center is violet. It is associated with the sense of compassion that comes from recognizing another as a reflection of yourself. The sense is the inner light that radiates from the eternal flame of sacred wisdom.

The mantra to nurture the seventh chakra is *Aum*.

So Hum Meditation

Every meditation technique offers something of value to the mind and body. We believe that procedures that quiet your mind allow you to glimpse the silent space between thoughts and help expand consciousness and heal the body. A very simple, effective, and easily learned meditation technique uses the breath along with a breathing mantra to quiet the mind and relax the body. If you are unable to receive personal instruction from a Primordial Sound Meditation teacher, the So Hum meditation described below will help take your awareness from a constricted to an expanded state of consciousness, aligning you with the Law of Pure Potentiality.

We recommend that you practice this technique for twenty to thirty minutes twice daily. We encourage you to perform it soon after awakening and again before dinner. Although some people find that if they meditate before bed they may have difficulty getting to sleep, you may find that by meditating at bedtime, you are able to turn off your mental turbulence from the day's activity and fall asleep easily after you have completed your meditation practice.

1. Sit comfortably where you will not be disturbed and close your eyes.

2. For a few minutes simply observe the inflow and outflow or your breath.

3. Now take a slow, deep breath through your nose while thinking the word *So*.

4. Exhale slowly through your nose while thinking the word *Hum*.

5. Allow your breathing to flow easily, silently repeating, *So . . . Hum . . .* with each inflow and outflow of your breath.

6. Whenever your attention drifts to thoughts in your mind, sounds in your environment, or sensations in your body, gently return to your breath, silently repeating, *So . . . Hum*.

7. Continue this process for twenty to thirty minutes with an attitude of effortlessness and simplicity.

8. When the time is up, sit with your eyes closed for a couple of minutes before resuming your daily activity.

Meditation Experiences

Although you may have a variety of experiences in your meditation practice, it is easy to classify them into a few basic categories.

Mantra Awareness

Your repetition of the So Hum mantra should be effortless. Silent repetition of the sound does not require clearly pronouncing it in your mind. Rather, have just a vague sense of the mantra, as a vibration, an impulse, or a subtle sound. Listen for its sound more than feel the pressure to articulate it. Whenever the mantra appears to be changing in its rate, rhythm, or pronunciation, allow it to transform without controlling the process.

Thought Awareness

The most common complaint that new meditators express is that they are having too many thoughts. Thoughts are a natural component of meditation, and it is not possible to forcibly stop thinking. There will be many times in every meditation during which your mind drifts off the mantra to thoughts. You may find yourself thinking about something that has happened in the past or something you are anticipating happening in the future. You may find yourself thinking about sensations in your body or sounds in your environment.

During this period of meditation, when you become aware that your attention has drifted away from the mantra, easily shift it back. Whether you are thinking about what you want for lunch, a movie you saw yesterday, an issue at work, or some profound cosmic realization, when you recognize that you have drifted off into thinking about something—anything—gently, and without straining, return your attention to the mantra.

SLEEP

If your body is fatigued when it is time to meditate, you may drift off to sleep. Don't fight the urge to sleep. Meditation is an opportunity for your body/mind to rebalance, and if it needs to rest, allow it to do so. When you awaken, sit up and meditate, using your mantra, for about ten minutes.

If you find yourself falling asleep in most of your meditations, you are probably not getting enough rest at night. Restful sleep is an important component of a balanced lifestyle. Be sure that you are exercising regularly, avoiding unnecessary stimulants during the day, and eliminating alcohol from your diet, particularly before bed. Try to be in bed with the lights off by 10 P.M.

PURE AWARENESS

As your mind quiets during meditation, you will experience moments when there is the absence of thoughts with the retention of awareness. We call this experience *going into the gap*. There is no mantra, and there are no thoughts. The mind has temporarily relinquished its attachment to time and space and is immersed in the eternal, infinite realm of pure awareness. This is the experience sometimes known as *samadhi*. With regular practice, the expansive awareness that you glimpse during meditation begins to permeate your life outside of meditation. The relaxation you gain while meditating extends into your activity. The ability to consciously experience nonlocal and local awareness simultaneously is the essence of yoga—established in a state of unity consciousness while being fully engaged in the world of forms and phenomena.

All of the Seven Spiritual Laws are in play during meditation. The process is governed by the Law of Pure Potentiality, which takes your mind to the domain of all possibilities beyond thought. Allowing mental activity to come and go without restriction expresses the principle of the Law of Giving and Receiving. Not indulging in the meaning of the thoughts that arise allows you to transcend the Law of Karma. The core principle of meditation is the Law of Least Effort, for the nonlocal field of awareness is also the domain of least effort. The state of nonlocal awareness, beyond thought, time, space, and causality, cannot be accessed through force. You utilize the Law of Intention and Desire by having the intention to relinquish your need to control, resist, or anticipate during the practice of meditation. The Law of Detachment is essential, for the only way to get to the field of unbounded awareness is by letting go. Finally, the Law of Dharma is active because it is the nature of the mind to seek ever-expanding realms of bliss and wisdom. It is the dharma of the mind to expand during meditation. Letting go and allowing the process to proceed innocently is the proven technique of going beyond thought and quieting the mind.

Attention and Intention Meditation

As you become adept at calming the commotion in your mind through meditation, you can enliven healing and transformation in your body through conscious attention and intention. As we've said, accomplished yogis can regulate basic physiological functions through inner techniques that focus attention and intention. You can learn to slow your heartbeat, raise your body temperature, and influence your circulation. Try this simple attention and intention meditation to convince yourself that your mind and body are intimately linked.

1. Sit comfortably, close your eyes, and take a slow, deep breath. Slowly exhale, releasing any tension you may be holding in your body. For the next few minutes, practice the So Hum meditation described earlier or Primordial Sound Meditation if you have been instructed in it.

2. Now bring your attention into the area of your heart. For a few moments, simply feel the sensations you are carrying in your heart and then for a few minutes consider all the things for which you are grateful. Acknowledge everything in your life for which you feel gratitude—the people, the love, the experiences, and the opportunities that make you the person you are.

3. Now take a few moments to relinquish any griev-
ances, regrets, or hostility you may be holding inside
you. Simply have the intention to release all toxic
feelings that are not nourishing to your heart.

4. Next, silently, like a mantra, repeat the expression,
*Thy will be done . . . Thy will be done . . . Thy will be
done.* Have the intention to surrender to whatever
you imagine or believe is the underlying intelligence
of the universe, be it God, Nature, Cosmic Order, or
any other concept that you have.

5. Now, with your attention in your chest, see if you
can perceive the throbbing of your heartbeat, as
either a sensation or a subtle vibration. Introduce the
intention for your heartbeat to slow down . . . slow
down . . . *slow down.*

6. Shift your attention to your hands and become
aware of your heartbeat in your hands. Have the
intention to increase the blood flow and warmth to
your hands.

7. Now direct your attention to any part of your
body that you believe needs healing and feel your
heart throbbing slowly in that area. If there is no
place in your body that needs attention, simply be
aware of your heart throbbing in your chest. Silently,
like a mantra, repeat the phrase, *Healing and transformation . . . Healing and transformation . . . Healing and
transformation.*

8. After a few minutes, bring your attention to your
breath, simply observing the inflow and outflow of
your breathing. When you are ready, slowly open
your eyes.

The Yoga of Meditation

The Upanishads tell us, "As great as the infinite space beyond is the space within the lotus of the heart." From the time of your birth, you have been called to explore the world outside of you. Meditation is the exploration of your inner world. Yoga encourages you to be as familiar with your inner world of thoughts, feelings, memories, desires, and imagination as you are with the outer world of time, space, and causality. When you can move through both the inner and outer domains of life with freedom and finesse, you fulfill the highest purpose of yoga.

6

Moving Energy
Pranayama and Bandhas

Why do you stay in prison when the door is so wide open?

—*Rumi*

Breath is the essence of life. You inhale for the first time shortly after arriving in the world even before your umbilical cord is cut. From that moment on you take approximately seventeen thousand breaths each day, which over a lifetime totals about 500 million breaths. In your final moments on this planet, you exhale for the last time; that breath defines the end of your life. Your breathing supports every experience you have from the time of your first inhalation to that of your last exhalation. Breath is life.

In yoga, the breath is intimately associated with prana, which translates from Sanskrit into English as "primordial impulse." Prana is the primordial life force that governs all your mental and physical functions. It is the vital energy that animates inert molecules into self-healing, evolving biological beings. It is the primary creative power of the cosmos.

Learning to regulate your prana to calm, balance, cleanse, and invigorate your body/mind is a powerful technique of yoga. Your breath integrates many layers of your life—your environment, your respiratory tract, your nervous system, your mind, and every cell in your body.

Regulating your breath enhances your physical, emotional, and spiritual well-being. It is the key to a healthy, vibrant life.

For most people, breathing is the only autonomic nervous system function that they can influence. Modern physiology divides the nervous system into two main components—the voluntary nervous system and the autonomic nervous system. The voluntary nervous system is active when you clap your hands, wave your arms, or use your legs to walk. It is responsible for activating the muscles that form the hundreds of facial expressions you make in a day, as well as those that control your speech. Although many of these functions occur with only minimally conscious intention, you have the ability to initiate and stop the use of these muscle groups at will.

The autonomic nervous system governs basic bodily functions, which you usually have no conscious ability to influence. These include core physiological functions such as heart rate, blood pressure, regulation of your temperature, the levels of hormones in your body, perspiration, and the movement of food through your digestive tract. Your autonomic nervous system also plays an important role in the regulation of your immune system. Modern neurological science suggests that most people are incapable of directly affecting these core physiological processes. They function on their own whether or not you are paying attention to them or attempting to alter them. Most people do not know how to influence their blood pressure, change the flow of their blood, reduce their sweating, or affect their digestive function.

Studies of yoga practitioners, however, have found that with practice, people can learn to consciously decrease their blood pressure, slow their heart rate, reduce their oxygen consumption, alter their circulation, and lower their stress hormone levels. Learning to influence these usually automatic functions is a different set of skills from those we use to ride a bicycle or kick a soccer ball, but it is one that you can master with a little practice. Learning to regulate your breath is the first step in discovering how to influence other essential involuntary bodily functions.

Left on its own, breathing does not require your conscious attention to consume oxygen or eliminate carbon dioxide. This is a good thing. Day and night, respiratory centers deep in your brain stem monitor the level of gases in your body and automatically adjust your breathing rate and depth. As anyone with asthma can testify, having to pay attention to breathing in order to get enough life-sustaining oxygen into your body is not desirable.

Every human being is capable of temporarily overriding autonomic control over breathing by speeding up, slowing down, or holding the breath. Conscious alteration of the usually automatic breathing process has powerful effects on your mind and body and provides a window into your ability to influence other autonomic functions. While you have your attention on your breath, you can modify it, but as soon as you relinquish conscious control, your involuntary nervous system resumes its authority.

Through the yogic practice of breathing exercises, known as *pranayama*, you can use your breath to influence your physical and mental states. A variety of techniques to relax or invigorate your body/mind are described in yoga. They are easily mastered and have prompt and powerful effects.

Pranayama Breathing Exercises

You can learn a lot about life by paying attention to your breathing. Right now, take a deep breath in and hold it. Feel the increasing discomfort that builds as you resist the natural impulse to let go. When it becomes too uncomfortable, release your breath and notice the immediate relief that you feel. Holding on to anything when it is time to let go creates distress in your body and mind. Now take a breath, fully empty your lungs, and hold your breath. Become aware of the increasing discomfort that develops when you resist something from entering your life that you are meant to accept. Notice the relief that you feel as you take your next breath.

Ingesting, absorbing, releasing, and eliminating—these are the key components of a healthy life and of natural, balanced breathing. When these basic functions are working well, you are able to absorb what you need and eliminate what you don't, resulting in life-sustaining nourishment and detoxification. When you take a bite of an apple, for example, you ingest potential nourishment, but the energy and information contained within the food do not become available to you until you've absorbed the basic nutrients through your small intestines. In every substance you ingest there are components that do not serve you, so a healthy digestive system releases the nonnourishing remains of the food into your colon. It is necessary to eliminate the residues of digestion on a regular basis for you to remain healthy.

These same steps are applicable on an emotional level. When people engage in emotionally powerful relationships, they often ingest more emotional energy and information than they are capable of digesting. To maintain a healthy emotional life, we must all selectively absorb those aspects of the emotional experience that are nourishing, while releasing and eliminating those components that, if retained, could be toxic.

The Law of Giving and Receiving is in continuous play during the practice of pranayama breathing exercises. Conscious breathing means focusing your attention on the perpetual exchange that is taking place between your personal body and the extended body of your environment. You exchange ten billion trillion atoms with your surroundings with every breath you take. The atoms you inhale every day have traversed the bodies of living beings across the universe and across time. Within you right now, you have carbon atoms that once inhabited the body of a cheetah in Africa, a dolphin in the South Pacific, a palm tree in Tahiti, or an Australian Aborigine. Ultimately, every particle in your body was stardust, created at the dawn of the universe. Your breathing is a continuous testimony to the Law of Giving and Receiving.

Conscious breathwork is also an expression of the Law of Least Effort and the Law of Dharma. In a healthy body, breathing is an effortless process, automatically speeding up or slowing down, becoming deeper or shallower with the subtlest shift in your body's requirements for energy. The oxygen you inhale supports the purpose (dharma) of every cell in your body, enabling each to exercise its unique talent while serving the wholeness of the physiology.

On both physical and emotional levels, pranayama breathing exercises clear the channels that enable you to effortlessly exchange your personal energy with the energy of the universe. Consciously directed, your vital energy can be used for creativity and healing. Pranayama breathing exercises are tools to help you channel your vital force in evolutionary ways that bring you higher levels of physical and emotional well being.

BHASTRIKA—BELLOWS BREATH

When you have a lot of energy moving through your body, you naturally breathe more vigorously. You spontaneously move more air when you are exercising or dancing because your body requires a greater quantity of oxygen to supply your energy needs. In the same way that invigorating action increases the depth of your breathing, you can consciously deepen your breathing, resulting in greater energy available to your body.

One of the most empowering breathing exercises in yoga is known as *Bhastrika*, which translated into English means "bellows breath." This is an energizing and cleansing breath. Although it is generally a very safe technique, it is important that you stay tuned in to your body during this process. If at any time you experience uncomfortable sensations or feel light-headed during the process, discontinue the Bhastrika for a few moments, then resume the exercise in a less intense manner.

Begin by relaxing your shoulders and practicing slow, deep abdominal breathing. After a few deep breaths, fully exhale, and then begin forceful complete exhalations followed by forceful deep inhalations through your nose at the rate of one second per cycle. The entire breathing movement should be from your diaphragm. Keep your head, neck, shoulders, and chest relatively stable while your belly moves in and out.

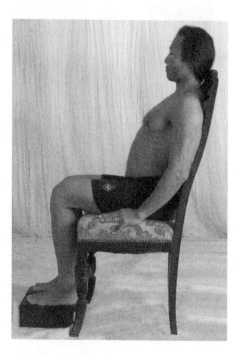

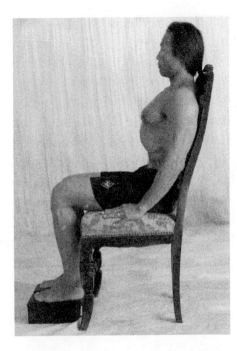

Start with a round of ten Bhastrika breaths, then resume normal breathing and simply observe the sensations in your body. After about fifteen to thirty seconds, begin the next round with twenty breaths. If you feel light-headed or experience tingling in your fingers or around your mouth, discontinue your deep breathing and simply observe your normal quiet breathing until the sensations completely subside, then resume the process.

After a pause of thirty seconds, perform a third round of thirty breaths. Again, suspend your Bhastrika breathing if you feel woozy. After the third round, simply witness the sensations in your body. For most people, this breathing exercise creates the experience of feeling energized and invigorated.

If you feel sluggish in the morning, perform a set of Bhastrika breaths and you will feel the clouds clear from your body and mind. You can also perform a couple minutes of Bhastrika during the day if you are feeling drowsy or lethargic. If you are trying to lose weight, performing Bhastrika several times per day will increase your digestive power and help your metabolism burn more intensely. It is generally not recommended that you perform Bhastrika pranayama close to bedtime as you may have difficulty falling asleep. Although Bhastrika clears the mind, it enlivens energy.

KAPALABHATI—SHINING BREATH

A variation of the bellows breath is *Kapalabhati*, which involves forceful exhalations followed by passive inhalations. Sitting comfortably with your spine in an upright posture, forcefully expel all the air from your lungs, then allow them to fill passively. The primary movement is from your diaphragm. Perform this movement ten times, then allow your breathing to return to normal and observe the sensations in your body. Repeat these cycles of ten movements three to four times. Like Bhastrika, Kapalabhati is a cleansing and invigorating pranayama.

DIRGHA—COMPLETE BREATH

Dirgha pranayama is a cleansing and balancing breathing exercise that shows prompt benefits. It involves consciously filling three different areas of your lungs. You start in the lower chambers, move up through the middle thoracic regions, and finish with the upper spaces. This breathing technique is a simple expression of the Law of

Intention and Desire. Simply by shifting your intention as to where to direct your breath you will notice a deeply relaxing and releasing effect.

Perform Dirgha pranayama either sitting upright or lying flat on your back. Both the inhalations and exhalations are through your nostrils.

For the first breath, inhale slowly and deeply, directing the air into your lower lungs by consciously using your diaphragm. When this is performed properly, your belly should inflate so you look like you are a little pregnant. As you exhale, deflate your belly, as if air were escaping from a balloon. Repeat this pattern several times, drawing the air into your lungs' lower chambers, maintaining smooth and rhythmic breathing.

After you are comfortable with this first step, begin bringing air into the middle section of your lungs. Start by filling your lower regions as before, then direct your inflow to your mid-lung region by opening your rib cage. You will feel your ribs expanding between your diaphragm and your chest. Inhale and exhale several times, filling both the bottom and middle areas of your lungs.

Finally, draw air into the bottom and middle regions of your lungs, then continue filling your upper lungs by breathing into your collarbones (clavicle). Practice the complete breath so your inhalation and exhalations flow in a smooth, continuous motion, sequentially directing your attention from your diaphragm to your ribs to your clavicle. Envision this deep, conscious breathing nourishing the organs, tissues, and cells in your body, enabling them to perform their vital functions effortlessly and in accordance with their dharma.

UJJAYI—SUCCESS BREATH

The pranayama technique known as *Ujjayi* can help settle your mind and body when you are feeling irritated, frustrated, or overheated. Although the origins of the word are unclear, one interpretation is "leading to success." This breath allows you to stay focused without generating unnecessary mental friction. Ujjayi creates a cooling influence at the back of the throat and has a balancing effect on the cardiorespiratory system.

To perform Ujjayi breath, take a slightly deeper than normal inhalation. On the exhalation, slightly constrict your throat muscles so as you breathe out it sounds as if you are snoring. The outflow of your breath is through your nose with your mouth closed. The result should be that you sound like Darth Vader from *Star Wars*.

Another way to get the hang of this practice is to first exhale the sound "haaah" with your mouth open. Now make a similar sound with your mouth closed, directing the outflow of air through your nasal passages. This should result in the desired breathy snoring sound. Once you have mastered it on the outflow, perform the same procedure on inflow, gently constricting your throat as you inhale.

Try shifting into Ujjayi breath whenever you find yourself becoming aggravated or upset, and you will notice a prompt soothing influence. Ujjayi is said to have a calming effect on the body while it helps the mind to focus. We recommend using Ujjayi while performing your yoga poses to help you stay focused as you move from one posture to the next.

Ujjayi can also be a useful tool during aerobic exercise.

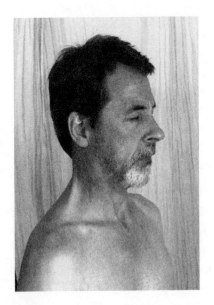

Olympic-level athletes have introduced Ujjayi into their training routines to enhance respiratory efficiency. Try using Ujjayi while performing your cardiovascular workout and see if practicing this breath technique reduces wear and tear on your body.

NADI SHODHANA—CHANNEL CLEARING BREATH

Nadi Shodhana means "clearing the channels of circulation" and is sometimes known descriptively as alternate nostril breathing. This pranayama exercise has a quieting effect and is very helpful in reducing mental turbulence associated with anxiety and insomnia. In Nadi Shodhana, you use your right hand to control the flow of breath through your nostrils. Your thumb is positioned over the right nostril, while your third and fourth fingers are over the left.

There are several different styles of Nadi Shodhana, all of which regulate the flow of air through your nasal passages. They differ according to how and when you alter the breathing pattern. The simplest procedure involves closing off alternate nostrils at the end of each inhalation. Inhale deeply, then close off the right nostril with your thumb, exhaling through the left. Smoothly inhale through the left nostril, and at the peak of the inflow, close off your left nostril with the third and fourth fingers of your right hand, exhaling through the right nostril. After full exhalation, inhale through the right nostril, again closing it off with your thumb at the peak of inhalation. Your breathing should be effortless with your mind simply witnessing the process.

Continue performing Nadi Shodhana for the next few breaths, following this pattern: Inhaling through the

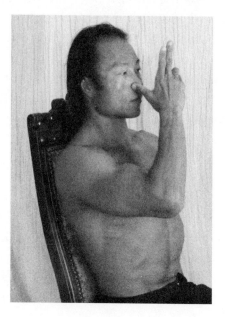

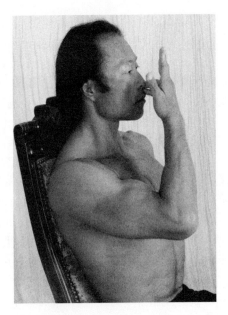

left nostril. Exhaling through the right. Inhaling through the right nostril. Exhaling through the left.

Nadi Shodhana has a relaxing effect on your mind and body. It can be useful to quiet your mind prior to beginning mantra meditation or when your mind is racing when you are trying to fall asleep. By softening the breath through Nadi Shodhana, you invoke a state of calm inner awareness.

Breathwork in Action

Become aware of your breathing throughout the day. If you find yourself in a tense or stressful situation, consciously take some slow, deep abdominal breaths through your nose and notice how your entire body relaxes. Practice Ujjayi breathing when you are walking or exercising and notice how it brings you back to your center. Use the Dirgha breath when you are feeling pressure and strain to circulate the life force throughout your body. Be conscious of your breath, and your awareness will stay centered in the midst of turbulence. According to yoga, this is the true value of pranayama.

THE BANDHAS—EMBRACING YOUR VITAL ENERGY

The word bandha means "to hold, lock, or embrace." These potent practices train you to direct your prana, or vital energy, to different centers of your body. Bandhas provide direct demonstration of the Law of Dharma as you witness the immediate reactions in your body to specific actions you take.

The basic principle with each bandha is first to accumulate energy in an area of your physiology, then release it. This process of building a force and then unleashing it discharges obstacles from the pathways of energy circulation. Like Traditional Chinese Medicine, yoga envisions the body/mind as a network of energetic channels through which life force flows. These pathways are known as srotas and nadis. Srotas are circulatory channels in the physical body, whereas nadis exist in the subtle body. Health and vitality are dependent upon life energy flowing freely through the physical and subtle biological passageways.

JALANDHARA BANDHA—CHIN LOCK

Sitting comfortably with your legs crossed in front of you, take a deep breath. While exhaling, bring your chin to

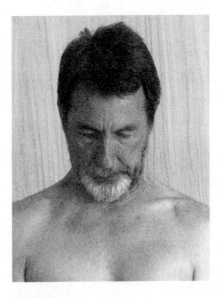

your chest. Pressing your chin into your chest, inhale against your closed throat so that no air moves but your chest rises up. Hold this position for ten seconds, then raise your chin and inhale normally.

The word *jalandhara* comes from two roots—*jala*, meaning "network," and *dhara*, meaning "upward flow." Jalandhara is designed to stimulate the network of nerves and energy channels in the throat. Energy stagnation in this region is associated with chronic neck pain, hoarseness, and thyroid imbalances. Jalandhara traditionally has been used to strengthen the thyroid, relieve neck stiffness, and enhance mental clarity.

UDDIYANA BANDHA—STOMACH LIFT

Sit comfortably with your legs crossed and your spine upright. Bend slightly forward. Placing your hands by your sides or on your thighs, bend slightly forward. Take in a deep breath and completely exhale, emptying your lungs as fully as possible. Make a motion as if you were about to take another inhalation, but instead lift your abdomen so that you are forming a hollow below your diaphragm. Hold this position for about ten seconds, then release and take a normal in-breath. Repeat this motion seven times.

This bandha activates the solar plexus energy center, which governs digestion and the ability to translate your desires into manifestations. Blockages in this region are associated with digestive disturbances and metabolic imbalances. Developing the ability to regulate energy in this area of your body ensures that you have access to your core digestive fire. When your fire is burning

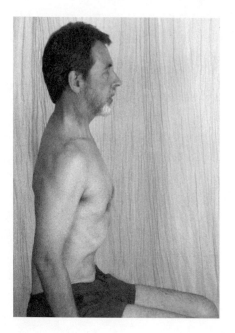

brightly, you are able to extract the nourishment you need from your environment and discharge toxins that inhibit the flow or energy in your body/mind.

Moola Bandha—Root Lock

Sitting with your legs crossed, bring your right heel as close to your groin as you can. With your eyes closed, begin contracting your anal sphincter muscles. Imagine as you are contracting that you are drawing your rectum upward into your abdomen. Hold this position for ten seconds, then slowly release while you exhale. Repeat this process ten times.

Moola means "root." The root chakra is the source of all energy in the body. Learning to regulate prana in this region will enable you to consciously direct your creative forces to the achievement of all your desires. Performing this bandha can help with a wide range of health conditions including hemorrhoids, urinary incontinence, and sexual function problems.

Pranayama exercises and bandhas bring your attention into your body and use your intention to move energy consciously. All success in life derives from this ability to consciously acquire, store, and release energy.

Learning to harness the power of your intention is the essence of the Law of Intention and Desire. The ability to direct your prana—your life energy—to eliminate toxicity from your body enables you to do less and accomplish more.

Not wasting your energy resisting the flow of your life force is the essence of the Law of Least Effort. Conscious breath work through pranayama and conscious energy management though bandhas teach you fundamental skills in governing the vital energy in your body. Pranayama breathing exercises and energy-regulating bandhas are fundamental practices that teach you how to manage your life energy efficiently and effectively.

The practice of yoga is practice for life. Learning these fundamental skills will serve you in all aspects of your life.

PART III

Yoga Practice

7

Consciousness in Motion
Yoga Asanas

Your body is precious. It is your vehicle for awaken-
ing. Treat it with care.

—Siddhartha Gautama

As you are reading these words, bring your attention into your body. Without moving, notice your posture. How are you sitting? Are your legs crossed? Are you in a comfortable position? Is there a part of you that is straining? Now make any adjustments in your position to enhance your comfort level. This is yoga. Changing your posture as a result of bringing your awareness into your body is the practice of yoga. The feedback loop is completed as changing your posture results in a spontaneous shift in your awareness.

Yoga is good for your mind and good for your body. Of the three important components of a balanced fitness program—flexibility, strength, and cardiovascular conditioning—yoga directly provides the first two and has the potential to enhance the third. Scientific studies on the health benefits of yoga have found that it can be useful in a wide range of conditions, including hypertension, asthma, depression, arthritis, heart disease, epilepsy, and cancer.

In the Seven Spiritual Laws of Yoga program, we have chosen postures to expand your flexibility, strengthen your muscles, and improve your balance. Each of the Seven Spiritual Laws enlivens the practice of yoga, while the practice of yoga enlivens your awareness of the Seven Spiritual Laws. Whether you are a beginning or an experienced yoga practitioner, this program will energize your body while taking your mind to a more expanded state of awareness.

Body Awareness Poses

We'll begin with postures that have the main purpose of enlivening body awareness. The word for "position" in yoga is *asana*, which means "seat." An asana is a position that you assume consciously. Yoga is the practice of consciously choosing the seat you assume. Although on one level, this means the physical position you place your body in, on another level, it implies that ultimately you choose every position in life in which you find yourself. Yoga then becomes a practice for making your choices more consciously so that the consequences of them are success and happiness.

As a human being, you have a built-in mechanism to

evaluate the choices you make in your life, which is by listening to the signals of comfort or discomfort that your body generates as you consider your options. This is the essence of the Law of Karma, which utilizes body awareness to make karmically correct choices. Learning to trust the feedback your body provides will enhance your ability to make karmically correct choices in life.

There are two important benefits of practicing yoga poses that enhance mind-body integration. The first is that yoga postures enable you to be more aware of the signals your body is sending so you can interpret them accurately. It is easy for human beings to be so immersed in their minds that they lose awareness of their bodies. The body is sending signals of what it needs, but the mind is too preoccupied to notice the signs. The practice of yoga enables you to reduce the mental background noise so you can pay attention to the messages of your body.

The second benefit of yoga is that regular practice of these poses will enhance your general level of physical and emotional comfort. If the background state of your body is one of chronic discomfort, it cannot be a reliable instrument by which you evaluate your choices. When using your body as an instrument for making choices, the subtle sensations of comfort or discomfort provide the guidance for right action. If your baseline state is disturbed, you will not be able to notice the shifts your body takes when considering different choices. Helping your body release obstacles that impede the healthy flow of life energy is a great benefit of practicing yoga postures.

Practitioners at all levels can perform these body awareness poses. It is important to remember that yoga is not a competitive sport. The goal of yoga is to enhance the connection between your body, mind, and spirit. The precise performance of a posture is of secondary importance to mind-body integration. Stay fully present as you move through these postures, gently moving into and then through your body's resistance.

PAVANAMUKTASANA—WIND RELIEVING POSE

Begin by lying on your back, allowing your awareness to float through your body. If you notice any area of tension in this resting pose, have the intention to release it. Now take in a deep breath and bring your right knee up to your chest. Grasp your leg below the knee with both hands and gently bring your chin to your knee. Hold this position for a few moments, breathing easily and feeling the sensations in your body. After several breaths, slowly straighten your leg, exhaling as you return it to the floor.

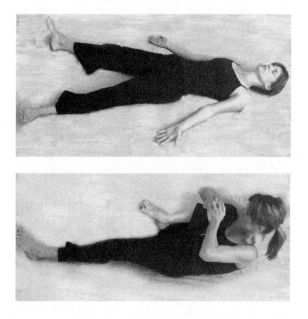

Repeat the pose with your left knee, bending it to your chest as you inhale, while raising your chin to your knee. Again, breathe easily for a few moments, then slowly lower your head and leg to the floor while exhaling.

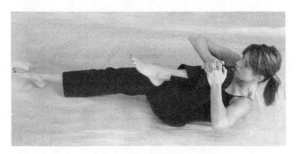

Now, while inhaling, lift both knees up to your chest, grasping both of your legs with your coupled hands. Hold for several moments, easily inhaling and exhaling and being aware of the sensations in your spine.

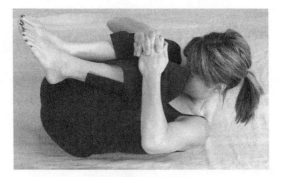

Now, holding both of your legs below the knees, gently rock backward and forward three or four times, then gently rock side to side several times.

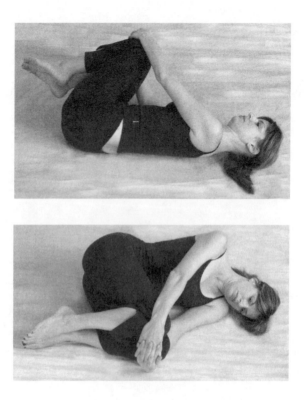

Returning to your back, gently begin bicycling motions with your legs. Placing your hands by your sides, extend first one leg, then the other. Inhale and exhale in rhythm with each leg extension. After about half a minute, return both legs to the floor.

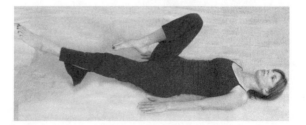

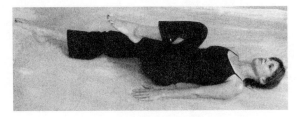

These are useful starting poses, for they begin mobiliz-ing energy in the body. According to Ayurveda, yoga's sis-ter branch of Vedic science, the vital airs of the body, known collectively as *vayu*, are the basis of all movement. Vayu governs the movement of thought, the movement of air, the movement of muscles, the movement of blood, and the movement of elimination. On a cellular level, it regulates the movement of DNA molecules, the move-ment of proteins, and the movement of hormones. Health results when vayu is moving harmoniously.

Vayu has a natural lightness, which naturally impels it to move in an upward direction. When vayu is disrupted as a result of stressful experiences, its job of eliminating toxins down and out from the body is impaired. Impair-ment in the elimination function of vayu results in energy stagnation, and the accumulation of subtle toxic-ity in the body. These wind relieving poses bring vayu back to its appropriate home in the pelvis so it can per-form its essential duty of moving toxins down and out of the body.

SARVANGASANA—SHOULDER STAND

While still on the floor, with your hands alongside your body, slowly raise your legs so they are perpendicular to the floor. Gently roll your weight onto your upper back as you elevate your hips, supporting them with both of your hands. Keep your upper arms and elbows on the floor. The back of your head and neck remain flat on the floor. Find a point of comfortable balance into which you can relax. Inhale and exhale slowly and deeply in this position.

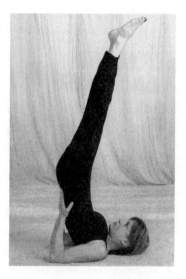

HALASANA—PLOW POSE

From the shoulder stand, gently lower your legs over and behind your head so you are touching the floor with your toes. If you cannot bring them all the way to the floor, lower them as far as you can. Place your arms alongside you, breathing easily, and feel the stretch in your spine and thighs. Bring your attention to your breathing and practice Ujjayi pranayama in this pose, audibly inhaling and exhaling with slightly constricted throat muscles.

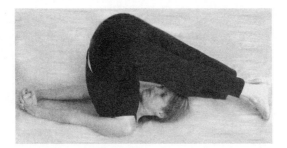

Slowly alternate between the shoulder stand and the plow pose three or four times. These two poses are beneficial for massaging the visceral organs and toning the thyroid gland.

Now slowly lower both legs back to the floor, resting comfortably on your back. Witness your breath while feeling the sensations in your body.

The shoulder stand and plow poses circulate energy up and down your spine. When you first try the shoulder pose, you may find that your center of gravity is in your hips and buttocks and you may have difficulty maintaining your legs over your head. With repeated practice, you will feel increasing comfort bringing your legs over your head and maintaining your balance with little effort. You may initially have difficulty flexing enough for your toes to touch the floor. After a few rounds of doing the shoulder stand alternating with the plow, it will be easier for you to obtain full benefit from both poses.

BHUJANGASANA—COBRA POSE

Roll from your back onto your stomach. Bring your legs and feet together with your toes slightly pointed. Place your palms beneath your shoulders, and while inhaling, gently begin raising your eyes, then your head, then your chest upward off the floor. As much as possible, use your spinal muscles rather than your arms to lift yourself up. Your lower abdomen should remain on the floor. Inhale as you rise and exhale as you lower yourself back down. Repeat this several times, then lower your chest to the floor.

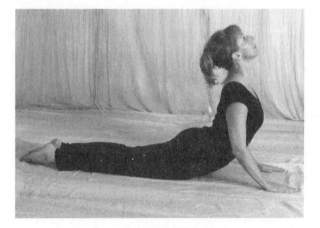

Salabhasana—Locust Pose

From your stomach roll onto your side. Make two fists side by side below your groin with your arms straight. Now roll back onto your stomach with your arms beneath your chest and abdomen. As you inhale, lift your right leg off the floor. Hold it for a few moments, then lower it while exhaling. Repeat this motion with your left leg. If you are able to perform this fairly easily, try raising both legs off the floor together, keeping your knees together. Inhale while you are lifting, hold for several moments, then lower both legs to the floor.

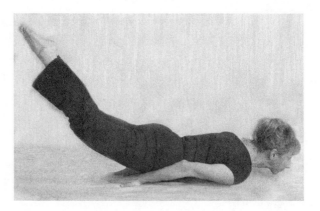

DHANURASANA—BOW POSE

Lying on your chest and abdomen with your forehead on the floor, tune in to your body, breathing easily. Now, slowly and deeply inhaling, reach behind you and grasp both ankles with your hands. Raise your head and chest off the floor while pulling your ankles up and toward your head. Lift your knees and thighs off the floor and look upward. Hold this position for several deep breaths, then gradually lower your legs and chest to the floor as you exhale.

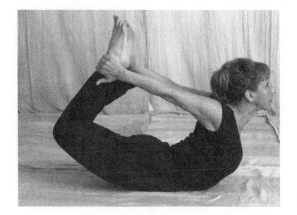

These three postures—cobra, locust, and bow—
extend your spine to increase backward strength and
flexibility. Modern life has a tendency to constrict the
spine with prolonged sitting at work and while traveling
in your car or in an airplane. As a result of this habit of
constriction, breathing becomes shallower and subtle
anxiety is experienced. Consciously extending the spine
counterbalances the restriction born of repeated flexion
and has a noticeable effect on both physical and emotional well-being.

These postures have a direct effect on improving
spinal health. Our spines consist of bony spinal vertebrae
separated by shock-absorbing disks. When you perform a
posture that extends the spine, the pressure is placed on the
back part of the vertebral body, which has the effect
of pushing the disks forward into their normal and
healthy position. The muscles that run along the spine are
strengthened through these poses, so that less weight is
borne directly by the disks. For people troubled by chronic
back pain due to bulging vertebral disks, the cobra, locust,
and bow poses help normalize the anatomy and reduce
back discomfort.

Janu Sirsasana—Bent Knee Forward Bend

Rolling to your back, assume an upright sitting position
with your legs out in front of you. Now, bend your right
knee and pull your foot tightly into your groin. Raising
both hands over your head, exhale while slowly flexing
forward at the waist, reaching forward to grasp your left
ankle or foot. If you cannot bend forward far enough to
reach your foot, hold your leg as far down as you can

without straining. In this position, use your breath to consciously release further into the pose, having the intention to relax with each exhalation. Hold this position, breathing deeply for several moments, then slowly release.

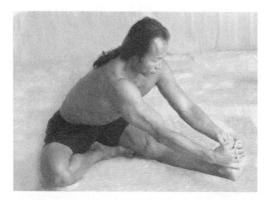

Repeat the pose with your left knee bent, flexing forward to grasp your right ankle or foot. Again, find your point of resistance, then introduce the intention to surrender, using your breath to release more deeply into the pose. Listen to the information your body is sending to you.

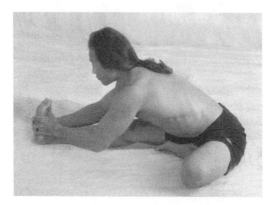

This posture provides a stretch to the hamstring muscles at the back of the leg. Opening these muscles through this pose translates into a more fluid gait.

PADMASANA—LOTUS MUDRA

Cross both legs in front of you, with your right ankle resting on your left thigh. If you can, bring your left ankle onto your right thigh, assuming a full lotus position. If you do not yet have the flexibility in your hips and legs to achieve a full lotus, remain in a half-lotus with your left ankle beneath your right thigh.

Now, flex forward at the waist until you are resting your lower abdomen on your thighs. Relax into this pose for several slow, deep breaths. Grasp your hands together behind you and slowly lift your arms upward, keeping them straight. Hold this position for ten seconds, breathing deeply, then lower your arms and slowly return to a sitting position.

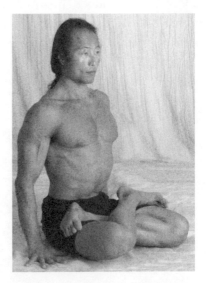

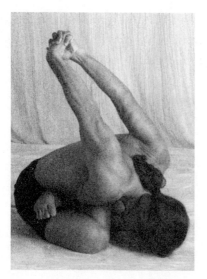

The classic lotus pose opens the pelvis and hips. Flexing forward in lotus increases the stretch in your hips and groin. Try switching the leg that is on top and notice how you are able to flex forward more easily each time.

UTTPLUTHI—UPLIFTING POSE

Continue sitting with your legs crossed in full or half-lotus. Place your hands flat on the floor on both sides of your thighs. Lift your entire body of the floor and hold for ten seconds. Then gently lower yourself to the floor.

This posture requires some upper body strength. At first, you may have difficulty raising your entire body. If so, allow your knees to remain on the floor while you raise your buttocks. Maintaining an upright pose, practice shifting your center point until you feel stable. If you practice the uplifting pose daily, you will begin lifting your entire body off the floor within two weeks. Remember

that the primary purpose of this pose is to bring your
attention inward, enhancing the communication between
the mind and the body.

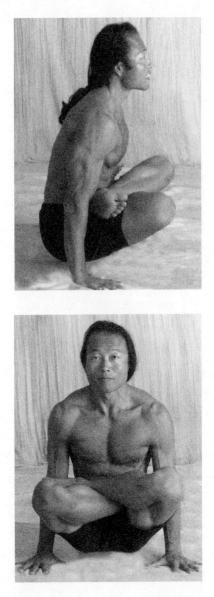

Balancing Poses

A healthy life is a life in balance. Yoga practice offers an opportunity for learning about dynamic balance. Maintaining mind-body balance provides the best platform to make karmically correct choices, enabling you to perform actions in the most efficient way. A life in balance is a life in dharma, for every action supports the evolutionary flow of life in which minimal resistance and maximum success are generated.

A balanced mind recognizes that we have control over the choices we make but not over the consequences of the choices. Putting your attention on the action rather than focusing on the fruits of action is the key to successful living. Yoga offers the opportunity to develop a balanced mind by bringing your attention into a pose while relinquishing your attachment to the outcome. Bringing balance into your body will awaken balance in your mind, just as bringing your mind into balance will assist you in finding physical balance.

The next set of postures is designed to awaken balance in your body and mind. Learning to maintain stillness in your body will help you cultivate stillness in your mind. At first, these balancing poses may be challenging for you, but if you practice them regularly, you will find them becoming easier each day, until you have mastered them. Notice how achieving stillness in your body spontaneously supports mental stillness.

Vrksasana—Tree Pose

Practicing this pose will help you develop the stability of a tree. Stand with your feet together and your arms resting comfortably by your sides. Close your eyes and become aware of your body's natural self-balancing movements. These subtle shifts in the activation of different muscle groups to keep you from falling are being orchestrated by an elaborate neuromuscular system. Balance centers in your inner ear and brain are continuously communicating with your postural muscles, helping you overcome the gravitational force that is trying to bring you down to the ground. Feel the Law of Least Effort and the Law of Dharma at work within you as you witness the perpetual adjustments that are occurring without your conscious input.

Now open your eyes and bend your right knee, bringing the sole of your right foot as high as possible onto your left thigh. Hold this position until you feel steady, then,

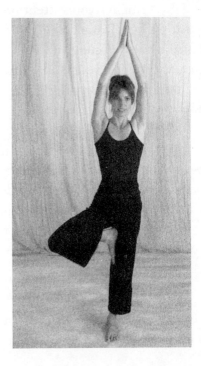

while balancing on your left leg, raise your arms over your head until your palms are together. Look straight ahead, breathing easily, and hold the pose until you barely require any adjustment to maintain your balance.

Lower your right leg to the floor, close your eyes, and again bring your attention in to your body, tuning in to your sense of balance and noticing any subtle changes that may have occurred as a result of holding the tree pose. Now, bring the sole of your left foot onto the inner aspect of your right thigh as high as possible, balancing on your right leg. Maintain stillness for about ten seconds, then return your left leg to the floor.

Practice the tree pose whenever your mind is turbulent. You will notice that as you bring your attention into the present moment, your body becomes still and your mind quiets.

Ekpadasana—One Foot Posture

Standing with your feet together, extend both arms in front of you so your palms are facing downward with your index fingers together. Balancing on your right leg, partially bend your left knee, bringing your left leg in front of you. Find your point of stillness while maintaining balance on your right leg.

Once you feel stable, slowly bring your left leg behind you while flexing at the waist until your left leg is extended out parallel to the floor. While you balance on your right leg, your arms remain in front of you with your palms facing the floor. Bring your attention to your breath as you find your center point of stillness.

Hold this pose for about ten seconds, then slowly return your leg to the floor and resume standing with

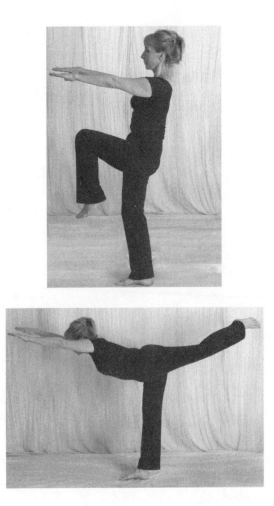

your arms at your sides. Close your eyes for a few moments, checking in with your body.

Repeat the posture with your left leg on the floor, first finding your balance with your right leg in front of you, then slowly bringing it behind you as you gently lean forward with your arms reaching forward. Slowly return to a standing position with both feet on the floor.

.   .   .

There will be times when your one-pointed attention locks in to a pose and body and mind come together. This is the essence of yoga. You are in present-moment awareness and there is effortless communication between your body and your mind.

TRIKONASANA—TRIANGLE POSE

From a standing pose, spread your legs apart so your feet are a little less than twice as wide as your shoulders. While inhaling, raise both arms straight up to shoulder height so they are parallel to the floor.

Turn your left foot 90 degrees outward, and bending from the waist, slide your left arm down your left leg until you can grasp your ankle just above your foot. If you cannot reach this far, grab hold of your leg as far down as you can reach. Bring your right arm up so it is straight and pointing directly toward the ceiling. Look up toward your reaching hand.

Hold this triangle posture, breathing deeply for five or six breaths, then gradually return to an upright position with your arms outstretched. Close your eyes and check in with your body for a few moments.

Repeat the pose with the opposite arm and leg. Turn your right foot outward 90 degrees and then slide your right arm down your leg, grasping your ankle while your left arm is pointing straight up. Take several slow, deep breaths before returning to an upright position.

The classical triangle pose enlivens both balance and flexibility. Use this pose to open your chest. Stretching while maintaining your balance is a great skill to develop in your yoga practice and in your life.

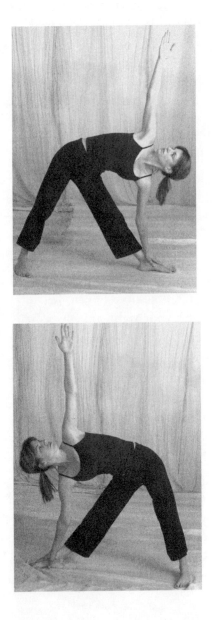

Dandayamana Konasana— Standing Angle Pose

Standing with your legs apart and your arms outstretched at shoulder height parallel to the floor, slowly bend forward, grasping your ankles with your hands. If you cannot reach as far as your ankles, grasp your legs as close to your ankles as you can. Now gently pull your head down toward the floor while you press your hips upward.

Hold this position for about ten seconds while slowly inhaling and exhaling, using your breath to surrender further into the pose. Slowly return to an upright position, take a few deep breaths, then repeat the standing angle pose two more times. Notice how each time you go into this posture it becomes easier to perform.

Flexion into this pose is initiated from your hips. You will feel stretching in your groin and lower spine. If you

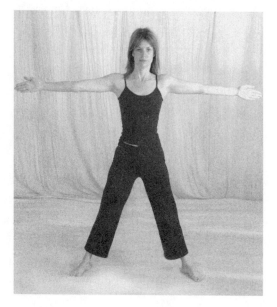

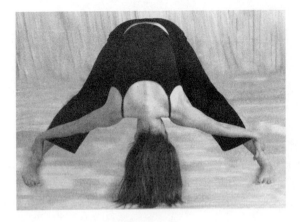

cannot grasp your ankles, try resting your hands on the floor in front of you and gradually walk them back toward your feet.

This pose allows you to see the world from a different angle, one of the benefits of yoga practice. Every person is a point of perspective, and it is easy for each of us to become attached to our particular point of view. Over time, this contributes to rigidity and judgment. Looking for opportunities to see the world from a new perspective nurtures flexibility in mind and body.

DANDAYAMANA DHANURASANA— STANDING BOW POSE

Stand with your feet together with both arms straight in front of you, palms facing downward. Bending your left knee, reach behind you with your left hand and grasp your left ankle. Flexing forward at the waist, pull your left leg upward as far as you can comfortably stretch it, keeping your right hand forward and parallel to the floor. You should feel a stretch in your thigh muscles. If you cannot maintain your balance without holding on, grab onto the back of a chair with your hand until you find your center. Hold this pose for ten seconds, then release your left leg and allow it to return to the floor.

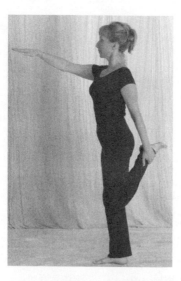

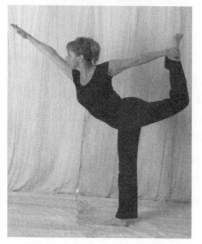

Repeat the pose on the opposite side, starting with your feet together and hands outstretched. Then reach back, grasping your right ankle with your right hand while you keep your left arm outstretched in front, palm facing downward. Hold this balancing pose for about ten seconds, then slowly return to a standing position.

The metaphor of the bow is used widely in yoga. To hit the target you are aiming at, you must first pull back to a still point that is full with potential. There is a classic Vedic story of an archery class in which Arjuna with his brothers and cousins are receiving instructions from the master archer, Drona. In a distant tree, Drona had placed a wooden bird onto which he had painted an artificial eye. He then asked each young man in succession to pull back an arrow but not release it until the student described what he was seeing. The first apprentice said that he saw the bird, the tree, the surrounding land, and the other students standing around him. Drona told him to put down the bow without launching the arrow. Each subsequent student responded similarly upon being asked the same question. When it was Arjuna's turn, his response was, "All I see is the eye of the bird." When asked by Drona, "Don't you see the bird, the trees, and the surrounding people?" Arjuna replied, "No, Guru, all I can see is the eye." At this response, Drona instructed him to release the arrow, which struck a bull's-eye.

The technology for success in life is first to pull back to a still, quiet inner place from which you can become clear about your goal, and then act with the full power of your intention. In yoga, the bow poses remind you to dive deep within yourself to find your quiet, unbounded state of awareness. When you act from this expanded domain of consciousness, your intentions will be powerful and success will be more likely.

GARUDASANA—EAGLE POSE

Most people find the eagle pose challenging when they first try it, but it usually can be mastered within a short period of time. Standing with your feet together, bend both knees, then shift your weight to your left foot. Cross your right leg around the front of your left until you can hook your toes inside your left calf muscle. You will need to keep your left knee bent to achieve this.

While your legs are wrapped and maintaining your balance, bend your right elbow and cross your left arm between your right arm and your chest. Place the fingers of your right hand onto the palm of your left hand and point

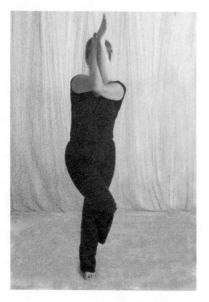

your fingertips to the ceiling. Hold this twisted pose for ten seconds, then unwind.

Repeat this balancing posture on the opposite side by shifting your weight to your right foot and wrapping your left leg around your right, hooking your left toes inside your right calf. This time, wind your right arm around your left so that the fingers of your left hand rest in your right palm. The opposite leg and arm are on top.

In Vedic mythology, Garuda is the eagle god—half bird and half man. He is frequently shown carrying Vishnu, the god who maintains the universe. Garuda is known as the destroyer of obstacles to the fulfillment of desires. Develop the focused attention and balance required to master the eagle pose and obstacles will dissipate from your life.

Practice these balancing poses on a regular basis and in addition to mastering the postures, you will find it easier to maintain your balance in all situations in your life. An underlying fundamental principle of yoga is the relationship between the individual and the cosmos, between the microcosm and the macrocosm. The skills gained during the practice of yoga translate into life skills. Everyone can benefit from greater balance in life.

Yoga in Motion— Salutations to the Sun

The twelve poses of the sun salutations offer an opportunity to enhance flexibility and strength while improving circulatory health. The set of postures has been described as the most complete exercise available, so if you have only limited time for yoga, the sun salutations are your best choice.

Through the twelve poses of the sun salutations, all major muscle groups and all major joints are exercised. These poses also massage and stimulate your major internal organs. These postures are designed to awaken the connection between your *agni*, or inner fire, and that of the sun. The word *agni* is the root of the English word *ignite*. When your agni is burning brightly, you are capable of digesting the energy and information you ingest on a daily basis, be it food, ideas, or emotional experiences. When your inner fire is weak and sputtering, you do not fully metabolize your daily life experiences. The residues of incomplete metabolism are stored in your body/mind, leading to fatigue and weakened immunity. When practiced along with following a healthy diet, a good daily routine, and the conscious avoidance of physical and emotional toxicity, the sun salutations are designed to kindle your inner fire so you can radiate the best of who you are.

The poses of Surya Namaskar represent the full experience of human life with all its highs and lows and ins and outs. Traditionally performed at sunrise and sunset, the postures represent the metabolism of the sun's energy into life energy. The sun is the source of all life on this planet. Ultimately we are beings of light, and the sun salutations acknowledge this primordial connection.

Performed slowly, the twelve poses encourage flexibility and strength. Performed rapidly, the sun salutes can provide a vigorous cardiovascular workout.

Along with each posture of Surya Namaskar is a mantra that awakens an aspect of the energy of the sun.

Say these sounds as you perform each pose and your mind will quiet and expand while you focus on the posture.

1. PRANAMASANA—SALUTATION POSE

Begin with your feet firmly planted on the ground in the salutation pose, inhaling and exhaling easily. Allow your attention to go inside and become aware of the current level of energy in your body. The mantra for the salutation pose acknowledges the unconditional life-giving power of the sun. This pose resonates with the heart chakra and the Law of Giving and Receiving.

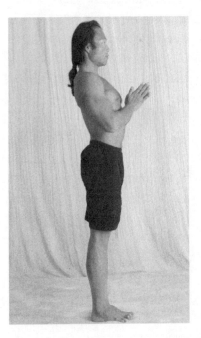

The mantra for the salutation pose is *Om Mitraya Namaha.*

2. HASTA UTTANASANA—SKY REACHING POSE

With your buttock muscles tightened, begin stretching up toward the sky while inhaling into the sky reaching pose. Stretch upward through your back, chest, arms, and neck. The mantra for this pose acknowledges the darkness-dispelling power of the sun. This pose awakens the throat chakra of expression and the Law of Detachment.

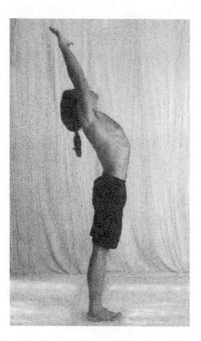

The mantra for this pose is *Om Ravaye Namaha.*

3. PADA HASTASANA—HAND TO FEET POSE

Next gently stretch forward while exhaling. Place your hands on the outsides of your feet, gently pressing your head toward your knees. Bend your knees as much as you need to in the hand to feet pose. In this forward flexion, you balance the extension of the previous pose. The mantra for this pose acknowledges the continuous movement of the sun, which induces daily and seasonal rhythms. It is associated with the creativity chakra and the Law of Least Effort.

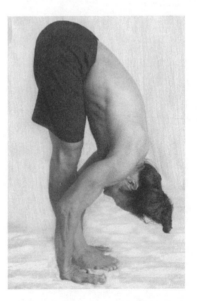

The mantra for this pose is *Om Suryaya Namaha*.

4. ASHWA SANCHALANASANA—EQUESTRIAN POSE

Now stretch back your right leg while looking upward, breathing easily in the equestrian pose. The mantra acknowledges the wisdom that dawns when light is brought onto a subject. It is associated with the chakra of intuition and the Law of Dharma.

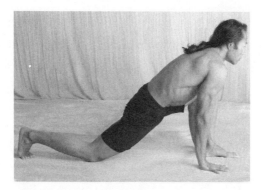

The mantra for this pose is *Om Bhanave Namaha.*

5. PARVATASANA—MOUNTAIN POSE

Next move into the mountain pose, with both legs
straight and together, raising your buttocks into the air,
stretching your arms. The mantra for this pose celebrates
the unlimited power of the sun. It is associated with the
throat chakra of expression and the Law of Detachment.

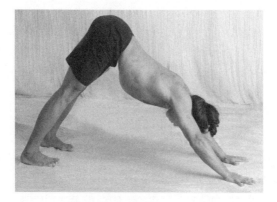

The mantra for the mountain pose is *Om Khagaya
Namaha.*

6. Asthanga Namaskar—Eight Limbs Pose

From this position, lower yourself gently to the ground, touching your forehead, chest, and knees to the floor, while maintaining the bulk of your weight on your hands and toes. This is the eight limbs pose. The mantra acknowledges the nourishment the sun provides to all living beings on earth. It is associated with the solar plexus (energy) chakra and the Law of Intention and Desire.

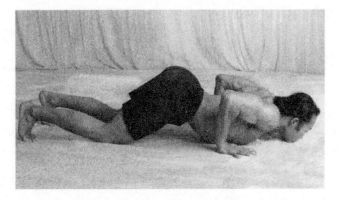

The mantra for the eight limbs pose is *Om Pooshne Namaha.*

7. Bhujangasana—Cobra Pose

Move directly into the cobra pose, rising off the ground using primarily your back and chest muscles. Do not overextend by pushing off with your hands. The mantra for this pose acknowledges the inner light that is reflected in the outer light of the sun. This pose resonates with the creativity chakra and the Law of Least Effort.

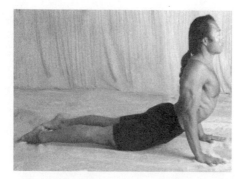

The mantra for the cobra pose is *Om Hiranya Garbhya Namaha.*

Return Cycle

The second half of the sun salutations is a retracing of the first half.

8. PARVATASANA—MOUNTAIN POSE

Return again to the mountain pose, this time introducing the mantra *Om Marichaya Namaha,* which acknowledges the transformational power of the sun. The Sanskrit name for black pepper is *marich;* it is believed to contain large amounts of solar energy.

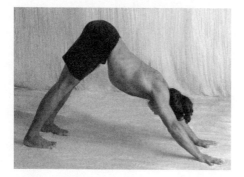

9. Ashwa Sanchalanasana—Equestrian Pose

Then move into the equestrian pose, this time with your left leg back. This mantra, *Om Aditya Namaha*, acknowledges the maternal nurturing aspect of the sun.

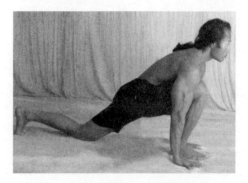

10. Pada Hastasana—Hand to Feet Pose

Continue the cycle by moving into the hand to feet pose, using the mantra *Om Savitre Namaha*, which acknowledges the stimulating power of the sun.

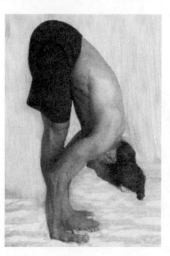

11. HASTA UTTANASANA—SKY REACHING POSE

Then move into the sky reaching pose, reciting the mantra *Om Arkaya Namaha*, which acknowledges the energizing aspect of the sun.

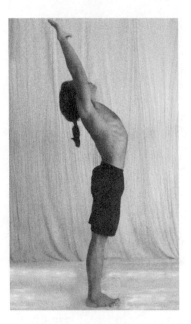

12. PRANAMASANA—SALUTATION POSE

Finally, return to the beginning by moving back into the salutation pose, using the mantra *Om Bhaskaraya Namaha*, which acknowledges the aspect of the sun that kindles the memory of wholeness.

The speed and vigor of the poses should be adjusted to suit your body type. It's best to start with a total of ten sets. As you become more comfortable, you can gradually increase the number. Breathe in harmony with the

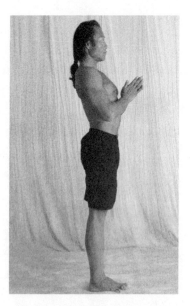

movements, so that you're inhaling each time the body is extended and exhaling each time you move into flexion. The postures are most beneficial when performed in a smooth, flowing, sequential manner.

According to yoga, if you do the sun salutations every day of your life, your mind will remain alert and vibrant and your body will be light and flexible.

Sun Salutations in a Chair

We believe that the sun salutations provide such benefit, and we have developed a modified version that can be performed in a chair. You can perform these modified sun salutations while riding as a passenger in a car on an extended road trip, sitting at your desk at work, or flying in an airplane. These poses relieve tension in your spine, enhance circulation, and ease soreness in your muscles.

Begin with the salutation pose by sitting comfortably in your chair with your spine upright and your hands at your chest, breathing easily.

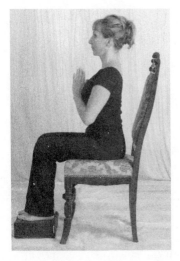

Inhaling, reach upward with both hands into the sky reaching pose, extending your spine.

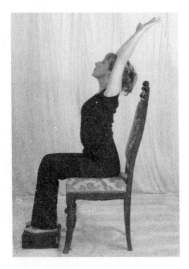

Bending forward into the hand to feet pose, lay your chest on your knees and allow your hands to rest alongside your feet. Exhale.

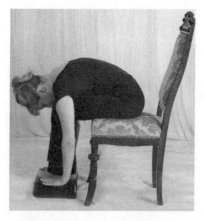

Arching your back into the extension pose (similar to the equestrian pose), pull your left knee up while looking toward the ceiling. Inhale.

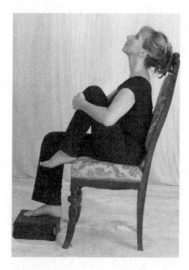

Partially exhale while bringing your chin down toward your left knee into the flexion pose (similiar to the mountain pose), gently rolling your back forward.

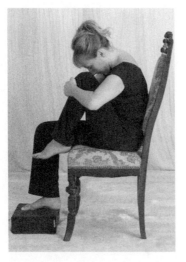

Again, flex forward into the hand to feet pose with your chest on your knees and your hands on the floor next to your feet. Exhale fully.

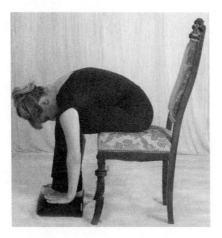

With your hands and arms remaining down by your legs, arch your back and neck into the cobra pose while inhaling partially.

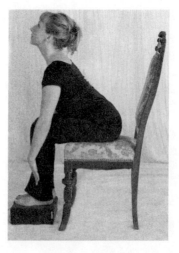

Now fully inhale as you bring your right knee up into the extension pose (similar to the equestrian pose) while extending your back in a gentle arch.

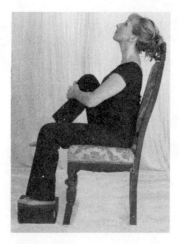

Partially exhale as you bend forward into the flexion pose (similar to the mountain pose), bringing your chin to your right knee.

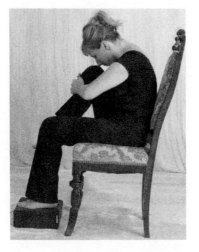

Fully exhaling, bend forward into the hand to feet pose with your chest on your knees, your neck flexed, and your arms alongside your legs.

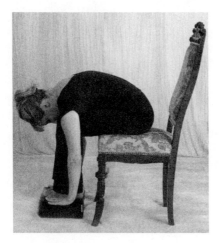

Stretch upward into the sky reaching pose, extending your spine while fully inhaling.

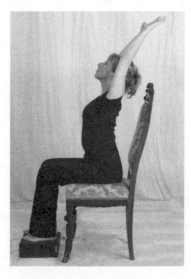

Return to the resting salutation pose with your hands at your chest, breathing easily.

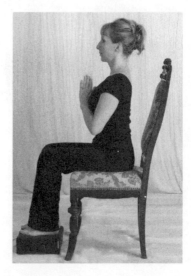

Energy-Opening Poses

Life energy flows up and down the spinal column. In yoga, the seven chakras are connected through three energetic pathways known as *Ida*, *Pingala*, and *Sushumna*.

Ida carries prana through the left side of the body, conducting feminine, lunar energy. When you are breathing through your left nostril, your Ida channel is open and receptive energy is active in your body/mind.

Pingala is the conduit for energy on the right side of the body, transmitting masculine, solar energy. When you are breathing through your right nostril, your active, goal-directed energy is more dominant.

Sushumna runs up the middle of the body, providing the connection between the root chakra at the base of the spine and the lotus center at the crown of the head.

When these channels are open, vital energy is able to flow freely. The vital energy rising up through the spine is known as the awakening of *Kundalini*, sometimes visualized as the uncoiling of a snake at the base of the spine. These final poses are designed to release congestion in the spine, enabling prana to nourish every organ, tissue, and cell in your body.

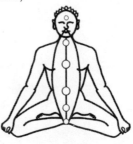

MATSYENDRASANA—SPINAL TWIST
(LORD OF THE FISH POSE)

Sit on the floor with your legs out in front of you. Bend your left leg and place your foot on the floor next to your right thigh. Place your right arm around your left knee and

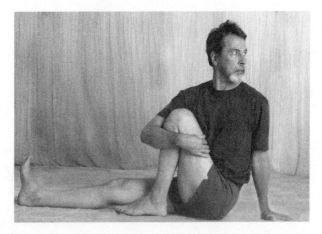

hold your right knee while twisting your spine to the left. Hold this position, breathing easily. With every exhalation, allow yourself to surrender into the pose.

Return to the midline and repeat the posture on the other side by bending your right leg and placing your right foot on the floor next to your left thigh. Place your left arm around your right knee while twisting your spine

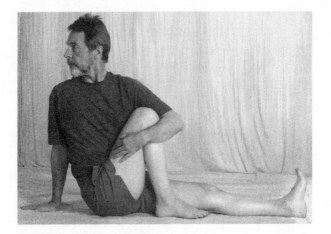

to the right. Again, breathe easily into the pose, using your breath to increase your flexibility. As you become more flexible, reach around and grasp the ankle of the foot that is placed on the floor. Hold for ten seconds, then return to center.

Close your eyes for a few moments and put your attention on your spine. Envision the life force flowing up from the base of your spine through your pelvis, into your abdomen, up through your heart, through your throat, between your eyes, and into your head. Imagine the thousand-petal lotus flower at your crown chakra opening. Activate the intention to live your life from a more expanded state of awareness as a result of energy flowing freely through your body.

According to Vedic mythology, Lord Shiva was instructing his consort Parvati on the essence of yoga on the shore of a remote island. Shiva noticed that a fish was listening intently to the discourse. Moved by the fish's concentration, Shiva gave a blessing over the aquatic animal, enabling it to assume a celestial form, whom Shiva named Matsyendra, or Lord of the Fishes. This pose is named in honor of this unusual sentient being.

CHAKRASANA—KNEELING WHEEL

From the spinal twist pose, roll your legs around so that you are on your knees with your feet close together behind you. Arch your back and grasp your right ankle with your right hand and your left ankle with your left hand. Raise your hips up toward the ceiling while allowing your head to relax backward. Breathe easily in this position for

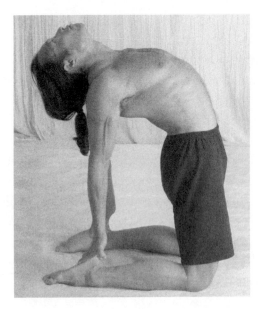

about ten seconds, then slowly lower your hips and raise yourself up, so you are again resting on your knees. Close your eyes and with your attention in your spine, envision energy moving up from your base to your skull.

This pose opens the pelvis and the spine, strengthening the neck and back muscles. Be conscious of your breath while holding this pose, having the intention to expand your chest with each deep inhalation while you stretch upward. In addition to forming the shape of a wheel (chakra), this pose activates each energy center.

VAJRASANA—DIAMOND POSE

Beginning on your knees with your body upright, gently lower yourself down until you are sitting on your heels. Rest in this position for a few moments, then lift yourself

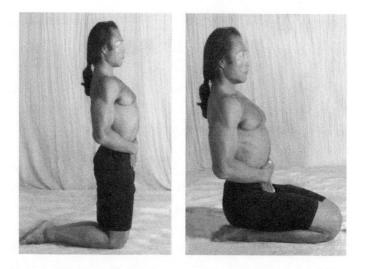

off your heels. Again allow yourself to settle onto your heels. Become aware of your breathing and allow yourself to relax more deeply with each breath. Activating the Law of Intention and Desire, envision energy freely flowing up your spine.

This is an energizing pose that awakens energy in the lower chakras. With practice you will see increasing flexibility in your hips, knees, and ankles. It provides benefits for people suffering with digestive disturbances and hemorrhoids.

The diamond is the precious gem that has the highest spiritual frequency representing purity and eternity. It has the ability to cut through almost everything else in the world. The diamond pose awakens the balanced state of mind-body integration that allows you to cut through ignorance with the wisdom of the infinite and unbounded field of life.

Matsyasana—Fish Pose

The fish pose provides a similar stretch to the spine as the diamond pose, but it is a little easier for most people. Not to be confused with the Lord of the Fish pose, matsya opens the chest, allowing for greater lung aeration. It is classically performed in a full lotus position, but it can also be done in half-lotus.

Sitting comfortably in the lotus posture, gently lower your back so you are lying on the floor with your crossed legs in the air. Place your palms flat on the floor just underneath your buttocks. While arching your back, lower your crossed legs to the floor. Resting on your bent elbows and forearms, continue arching your back until the crown of your head is on the floor. Breathe easily while holding this position for fifteen seconds. Then lower your back to the floor and slowly uncross your legs.

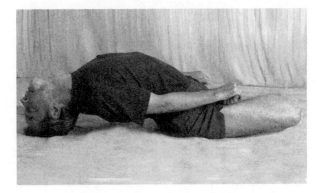

If you are unable to get into a full lotus, you can perform a simpler modification of the fish pose. Lying on your back, bend your knees and bring your heels as close as you can to your buttocks. Bear your weight on your elbows and forearms while arching your back until you are able to rest the top of your head on the floor. Feeling the stretch in your neck and back, hold this posture for fifteen seconds, then slowly lower your back and then your legs to the ground.

Balasana—Child's Pose

Kneeling on the floor, overlap your big toes and sit on your heels. Separate your knees and slowly bend forward until you are resting your body between your thighs. Lay your hands on the floor alongside your torso, palms up, and release your shoulders toward the floor. Rest your forehead on the floor and breathe easily.

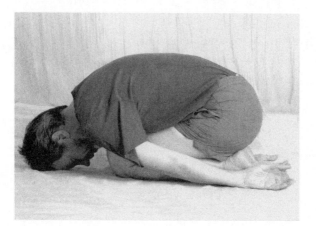

The child's pose is a comfortable resting posture that allows you to quiet your mind as your body settles into deeper relaxation. In many ways it is the asana equivalent of the fetal position. Bring the Law of Least Effort into your awareness as you surrender into the child's pose, feeling the sense of inner safety that this posture generates.

Children are flexible and have an amazing capacity to adapt to changing situations even as they have limited ability to control the course of their own lives. Despite the fact that they are subject to the will of adults who direct their lives, children are able to find joy in their present moment. Flexibility and adaptability are valuable qualities that yoga can cultivate to reestablish some of the resiliency of youth.

Carl Jung once said that as children we have unconscious perfection. As adults we become conscious of our imperfection. Finally, with wisdom we achieve a state of conscious perfection.

The child's pose provides an opportunity to quiet the mind, relax the body, and celebrate the state of conscious perfection. Whenever you feel that the demands of the world are becoming too burdensome, assume this pose and allow the Law of Least Effort and the Law of Detachment to spontaneously awaken within you.

Yoga in Action

The human body is designed for movement. When you are able to move freely, effortlessly, and in harmony with your environment, you experience joy and vitality on all levels of life. This is the highest expression of the Law of Dharma—established in a state of expanded inner awareness, you perform activity with dynamic ease. The regular practice of yoga enables you to expand your limitations. As the body becomes more flexible, the mind becomes more flexible. As the body gains strength, the mind gains strength. As you learn to maintain a centered state of balance physically, you spontaneously feel more centered and balanced mentally and emotionally.

According to the Seven Spiritual Laws, you have the potential to create a magnificent life filled with wisdom, success, and love. The creative cauldron of Pure Potentiality resides within you in the domain of silence at the source of your mind and body. You can access this field through the stillness cultivated in your practice of yoga.

Joy in life flows from the effortless giving and receiving that derives from a deep connectedness to spirit. Every breath and movement you perform in yoga reminds you to allow vital energy to flow freely between your personal body and your extended body, spontaneously awakening the Law of Giving and Receiving in your life.

The Law of Karma reminds you that every action has its reaction. Performing actions consciously in your yoga practice ensures that the reactions generated by your choices are more likely to be evolutionary for you and for those around you.

Opening to the possibility that you don't have to struggle so hard to achieve your goals is the essence of the Law of Least Effort. Every practice session of yoga reminds you of this basic principle. If you force yourself into a posture, you will almost certainly pay the price the next day of decreased rather than increased flexibility. Yoga is practice for living life with finesse.

Your intentions orchestrate their fulfillment. Become aware of the Law of Intention and Desire in your yoga practice as you move into every posture. Introduce your intention and then let go. It is this paradoxical coexistence of the Law of Intention and Desire along with the

Law of Detachment that taps into the power of nature to support your deepest aspirations.

Every moment is as it should be. From the beginning of time and space, the universe has been unfolding as through unfathomable multidimensional coincidences. Struggling against this moment is struggling against the entire universe.

The practice of yoga awakens the Law of Dharma in your life by teaching you to feel your way. Your body is capable of calculating the most evolutionary choices available to you at every moment. You simply need to be able to listen to the signals it is sending you in its desire to support your happiness and health.

A yogic practice eliminates the static in the communication lines between your mind and body. The clarity, flexibility, balance, strength, and centered awareness that you cultivate while practicing your postures will serve you well throughout your day and throughout your life.

8

The Seven Spiritual Laws of Yoga Session

*We have what we seek. It is there all the time, and
if we give it time it will make itself known to us.*
                              —Thomas Merton

You now have all the components for the complete
Seven Spiritual Laws of Yoga program. The full
program is designed to take your body and mind from a
state of deep silence through conscious breathing into
positions that enhance flexibility, strength, and balance.
Vigorous performance of the sun salutations will also
help condition your cardiovascular system, while energy-
governing exercises enable you consciously to channel
your vital force. After performing the physical techniques, we encourage you to spend a few minutes bringing
the spiritual law of the day into your awareness so it

remains lively throughout the day. The major facets of the program include:

Pranayama breathing exercises

Meditation

Flexibility postures

Balance postures

Sun salutations

Bandhas

Energy-opening postures

The spiritual law of the day

As a sign of commitment to the well-being of your body, mind, and soul, spend some time every day practicing yoga. When practicing on your own, an ideal session is as follows:

Pranayama (5 to 10 minutes)

Begin with five to ten minutes of pranayama breathing exercises. Start with several rounds of Bhastrika, or bellows breath, to clear your body of toxins. Then perform three or four Dirgha breaths, bringing air sequentially into your lower, middle, and upper lung spaces. Next, shift into Ujjayi breathing for several minutes, slowly inhaling and exhaling with a slight contraction of your throat muscles. Finally, move into Nadi Shodhana, or alternate nostril breathing. Partially close your eyes as you perform Nadi Shodhana to draw your attention inward. Depending upon how much time you have available, spend five to ten minutes performing your breathing exercises.

Bhastrika (1 to 2 minutes)—bellows breath

Dirgha (1 to 2 minutes)—complete breath

Ujjayi (1 to 2 minutes)—success breath

Nadi Shodhana (2 to 4 minutes)—clearing breath

So Hum Meditation (10 to 30 minutes)

After clearing the subtle channels of circulation with your pranayama breathing exercises, you are ready to take your attention to a more expanded state of awareness through meditation. Close your eyes completely and simply become aware of your thoughts for a few moments, then sequentially bring your attention to each of the seven chakras, audibly intoning the mantra for each energy center.

After awakening these junction points between the mind and the body, it is time to calm your mind. Begin your silent meditation by practicing breathing awareness using the So Hum mantra or any other mind-quieting procedure you have learned. We encourage you to learn Primordial Sound Meditation from a qualified instructor.

Meditation ideally is practiced for twenty to thirty minutes. If you cannot accommodate this full-time, allow for at least ten minutes of meditation during your yoga practice. Always take a few minutes at the end of your meditation to gently stretch and move before opening your eyes.

Flexibility Postures (10 to 20 minutes)

Having cleared your channels and quieted your mind, you are now ready to begin moving energy consciously through the yoga poses. Begin with the flexibility poses, taking a minute or two to move into each of the nine postures.

1. PAVANAMUKTASANA—WIND RELIEVING POSE

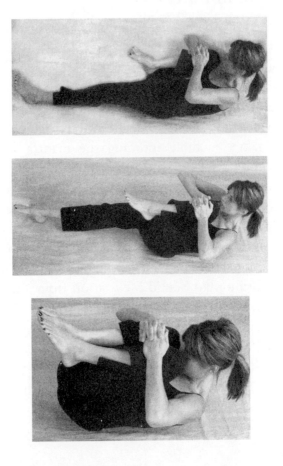

2. SARVANGASANA—SHOULDER STAND

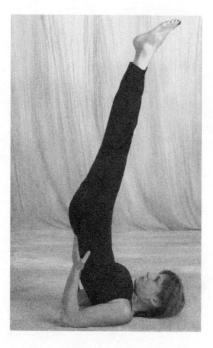

3. HALASANA—PLOW POSE

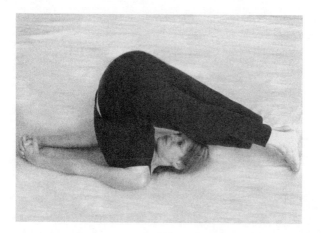

4. Bhujangasana—Cobra Pose

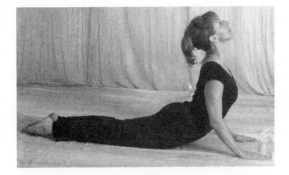

5. Salabhasana—Locust Pose

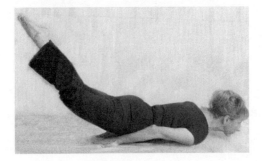

6. Dhanurasana—Bow Pose

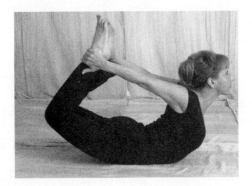

7. Janu Sirasana—Bent Knee Forward Bend

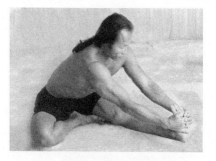

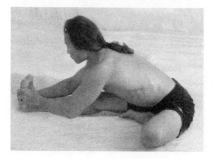

8. Padmasana—Lotus Flexion

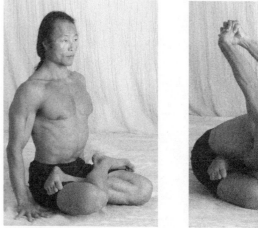

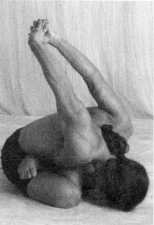

9. Uttpluthi—Uplifting Pose

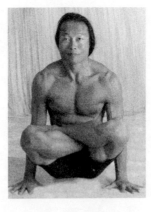

Balancing Postures (5 to 10 minutes)

With enhanced flexibility, you naturally become better at maintaining your balance. Spend about a minute in each of the six balancing poses, noticing how your inner mental turbulence quiets as you find your physical center.

1. Vrksasana—Tree Pose

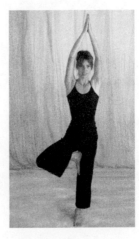

2. Ekpadasana—One Foot Pose

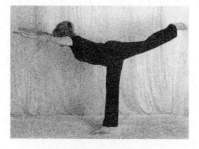

3. Trikonasana—Triangle Pose

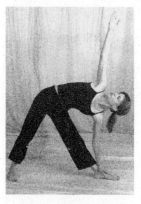

4. Dandayamana Konasana— Standing Angle Pose

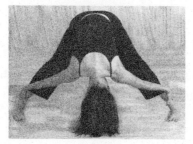

5. DANDAYAMANA DHANURASANA— STANDING BOW POSE

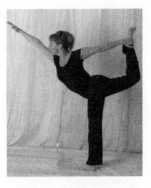

6. GARUDASANA—EAGLE POSE

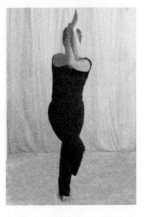

Sun Salutations (5 to 20 minutes)

The flowing sequential movements of the sun salutations can be performed slowly or energetically. In the context of this sequence, we recommend you perform your twelve postures briskly. Begin with six sets, which may take you about five minutes, gradually progressing until you are performing sun salutations for fifteen to twenty minutes. In addition to stretching your muscles and joints, you will exercise your heart and improve your circulation.

1. SALUTATION POSE

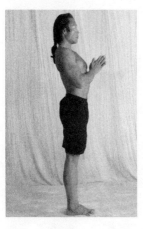

2. SKY REACHING POSE

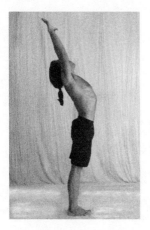

3. HAND TO FEET POSE

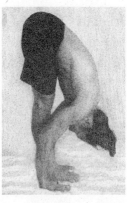

4. EQUESTRIAN POSE

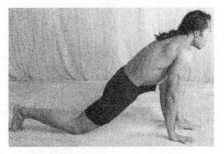

5. MOUNTAIN POSE

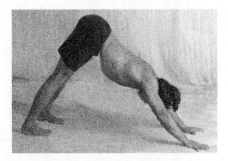

6. EIGHT LIMBS POSE

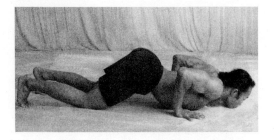

7. COBRA POSE

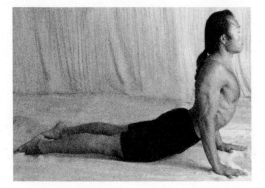

8. MOUNTAIN POSE

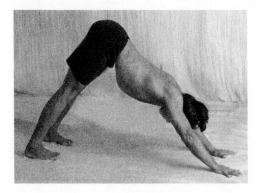

9. Equestrian Pose

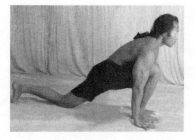

10. Hand to Feet Pose

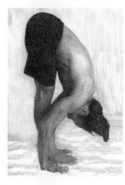

11. Sky Reaching Pose

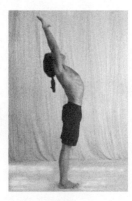

12. SALUTATION POSE

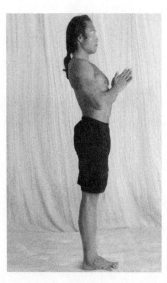

Bandhas (2 to 5 minutes)

It is useful at this stage to perform your energy-governing techniques. Begin with the chin lock bandha, in which you fully exhale, flexing your head forward, and then inhale against a closed throat. Release after several seconds, then begin the stomach-lift bandha, in which you raise your stomach using your abdominal and diaphragm muscles. Finally, awaken the energy at the base of your spine by performing the root bandha, contracting your sphincter muscles.

Jalandhara bandha (1 minute)—chin lock

Uddiyana bandha (1 minute)—stomach lift

Moola bandha (1 minute)—root lock

Energy-Opening Postures (5 to 10 minutes)

Ending your asana set with these four energy-opening poses enables you to channel vitality into all aspects of your life. Perform each of these postures with conscious awareness, allowing the life force to flow effortlessly into every organ, tissue, and cell of your body.

1. MATSYENDRASANA—SPINAL TWIST

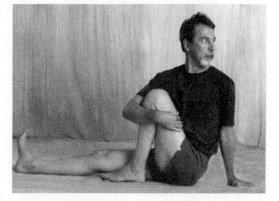

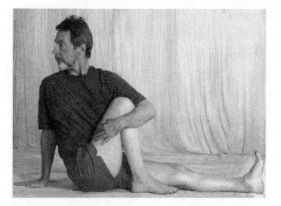

2. CHAKRASANA—KNEELING WHEEL POSE

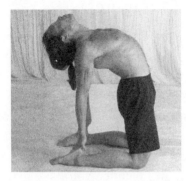

3. SUPTAVAJRASANA—DIAMOND KNEELING

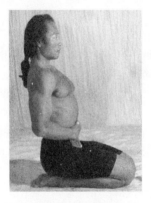

4. BALASANA—CHILD'S POSE

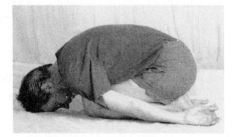

Activate the Spiritual Law of the Day (5 minutes)

At the end of your program, lie on your back with your arms at your sides and allow your total awareness to be in your body. Enjoy the sensations generated by consciously moving the life force through you.

Bring the spiritual law of the day into your awareness, committing to enlivening it by attending to the three activating intentions. As a result of the expanded awareness, flexibility, and balance you have generated in your practice, the law of the day will spontaneously support you in the fulfillment of your deepest desires.

Spiritual Law of the Day

Day	Spiritual Law	Activating Intentions
Sunday	Pure Potentiality	1. Cultivate stillness 2. Commune with nature 3. Practice nonjudgment
Monday	Giving and Receiving	1. Practice breath awareness 2. Cultivate gratitude 3. Acknowledge your needs
Tuesday	Karma (or Cause and Effect)	1. Witness your choices 2. Consider the consequences 3. Listen to your heart
Wednesday	Least Effort	1. Practice acceptance 2. Accept responsibility 3. Be defenseless
Thursday	Intention and Desire	1. Be clear of your intentions 2. Trust the outcome 3. Practice present moment awareness

Day	Spiritual Law	Activating Intentions
Friday	Detachment	1. Practice detachment 2. Embrace uncertainty 3. Surrender to the field of pure potentiality
Saturday	Dharma (or Purpose in Life)	1. Attend to your silent witness 2. Acknowledge your talents 3. Serve others

Prioritizing

If you spend some time in each stage of this program, you can spend as little as three-quarters of an hour or almost two hours in your practice. Decide for yourself the pace and intensity that you can execute. The time you spend will yield rewards physically, emotionally, and spiritually. Commit to this program for one month and you will be a yogi for life.

Conclusion

From here, what you see you become.

—Patanjali

According to Indian philosophy, yoga is the system of gaining knowledge through direct experience. A chemist may understand the molecular basis of a strawberry. A geneticist may understand the DNA sequences that underlie different varieties of strawberries. A botanist may know the precise soil and water requirements for a strawberry plant to thrive. A yogi knows the strawberry by taking a bite.

Yoga declares that you can understand reality by consciously experiencing the different layers of your life—physical, mental, and spiritual. By tuning in to the sensations of your body, you can understand the workings of physiology. By listening to your inner dialogue, you can understand the nature of the mind. By going beyond your body and your mind, you can directly experience your essential spiritual core.

Yoga encourages you to expand your sense of self so you can solve the challenges that arise in your life. Each of us is a heroic character on the battlefield of life. The perennial story of life is depicted in the Indian classic, the *Bhagavad Gita*, in which the forces of good and the forces of evil find residence in two clans of the same family. The Pandava clan, led by Arjuna, represents right action in accordance with natural law. The Kauravas, headed by Duryodhana, represent action performed with limited awareness resulting in outcomes that cause suffering to those affected by the choices made. The *Bhagavad Gita* begins with these two opposing forces on the battlefield of life preparing for massive conflict.

Both Arjuna and Duryodhana ask Lord Krishna, representing the state of expanded consciousness, for support. Krishna offers one leader the use of his army while the other gets him as his personal charioteer. Duryodhana gets to choose first and takes the army, believing that the power of might will provide him the greatest benefit. The power of expanded awareness in the form of Krishna goes to Arjuna.

Krishna takes Arjuna above the battlefield, where Arjuna confesses his confusion about what to do. On the one hand, he believes it is his duty to fight his relatives who have created havoc in the world. On the other hand, he feels tremendous compassion for the uncles and cousins who have played important roles in his life. Arjuna is paralyzed by his inner battle. The tremendous value of yoga is the depiction of this classic conflict between heart and mind that each of us faces during our lives.

While time is suspended, Krishna teaches Arjuna the essence of yoga, telling him that good and evil, pleasure and pain, and loss and gain are two sides of the same coin of life. The solution that yoga offers is to go beyond the realm of duality and become established in the state of being that is beyond time, space, and causality. Once rooted in this connection to spirit, Arjuna is exhorted to enter into battle to rebalance the forces of nature.

Krishna tells Arjuna, "Go beyond the realm of good and evil where life is dominated by beginnings and endings. Enter into the domain of yoga, where all duality finds its unity. Established in unity, perform activity that supports dharma."

This is the ultimate purpose of a yoga practice. Yoga takes you into the realm of Pure Potentiality, where anything is possible. It awakens the Law of Giving and Receiving as you become aware of the continuous exchange of your life energy with the life energy of the universe. Flexing and extending through your poses, you express the Law of Karma as you recognize that every action generates a proportionate reaction. The Law of Least Effort becomes lively as you surrender into each posture, releasing rather than forcing your way into a position. Combining the Law of Intention with the Law of Detachment, yoga demonstrates that introducing your desire and allowing nature to orchestrate its fulfillment maximizes achievement while minimizing strain. Finally, moving gracefully, sensitively, and consciously is the technology of living the Law of Dharma in which your actions have a positive effect on you and your environment.

Any reason for practicing yoga is a good reason. Enhancing flexibility and releasing stress are as noble a purpose for performing yoga as the awakening of spirituality. This is the great gift of yoga—it serves and nourishes us at every level of our being and spontaneously contributes to greater well-being in all domains of life.

The practice of yoga is worthy of your valuable time and attention. Yoga will help you discover gifts within yourself that have remained unopened since your childhood—gifts of peace, harmony, laughter, and love.

Recommended Reading

By Deepak

The Seven Spiritual Laws of Success. San Rafael, Calif.: Amber-Allen Publishing, 1994.

How to Know God. New York: Harmony Books, 2000.

The Spontaneous Fulfillment of Desire. New York: Harmony Books, 2003.

By David

The Wisdom of Healing. New York: Three Rivers Press, 1997.

Return to Wholeness. New York: John Wiley & Sons, 1999.

Vital Energy. New York: John Wiley & Sons, 2000.

By Our Teachers

Aurobindo, Sri. *Integral Yoga: Sri Aurobindo's Teaching and Method of Practice*. Twin Lakes, Wisc.: Lotus Press, 1993.

Frawley, David. *Yoga and Ayurveda*. Twin Lakes, Wisc.: Lotus Press, 1999.

Iyengar, B. K. S. *Light on the Yoga Sutras of Patanjali*. London: Thorsons, 1996.

Maharaj, Nisargadatta. *I Am That: Talks with Sri Nisargadatta*. Durham, N.C.: Acorn Press, 1973.

Osho. *Meditation: The First and Last Freedom*. New York: St. Martin's Press, 1996.

Saraswati, Swami Satyananda. *Asana Pranayama Mudra Bandha*. Munger, Bihar, India: Yoga Publications Trust, 1996.

Venkantesananda, Swami. *The Concise Yoga Vasishta*. Albany, N.Y.: SUNY Press, 1985.

Viveka-Chudamani. *Shankara's Crest Jewel of Discrimination*. Hollywood, Calif.: Vedenta Press, 1978.

Index

Page numbers in italics refer to illustrations.

The Chopra Center

A PLACE OF HEALING AND TRANSFORMATION

Fulfilling a lifelong dream of creating an environment that focuses on enhancing health and nourishing the human spirit, Deepak Chopra, M.D., and David Simon, M.D., opened the Chopra Center For Well Being in 1994. Centrally located on the grounds of the La Costa Resort & Spa, the center offers a wide variety of individual and group programs in mind/body medicine, healing therapies, and personal development. Integrating the best of western and natural healing traditions, the Chopra Center provides a fresh approach to modern health-care needs. Under the direction of Drs. Chopra and Simon, guests can actively participate in programs, workshops, and seminars that physically, emotionally, and spiritually nourish, cleanse, and uplift.

Guests at the Chopra Center can avail themselves of the world-class Chopra Center Spa, where ancient mind/body holistic techniques are blended with cutting-edge natural treatments to awaken, rejuvenate, and heal. Designed by Drs. Chopra and Simon, the Chopra Center's spa treatments are founded in the perennial principles of Ayurveda—the five-thousand-year-old healing system of India.

For more information on the Chopra Center's Seven Spiritual Laws of Yoga program and all of our workshops, seminars, services, and products for healing and transformation, please visit us at www.chopra.com, e-mail us at yoga@chopra.com, or call us at (888) 424-6772.